Plastic Surgery for Men

Editors

DOUGLAS S. STEINBRECH
ALAN MATARASSO

CLINICS IN
PLASTIC SURGERY

www.plasticsurgery.theclinics.com

April 2022 • Volume 49 • Number 2

ELSEVIER

1600 John F. Kennedy Boulevard • Suite 1800 • Philadelphia, Pennsylvania, 19103-2899

http://www.theclinics.com

CLINICS IN PLASTIC SURGERY Volume 49, Number 2
April 2022 ISSN 0094-1298, ISBN-13: 978-0-323-89742-6

Editor: Stacy Eastman
Developmental Editor: Jessica Nicole B. Cañaberal

Clinics in Plastic Surgery (ISSN 0094-1298) is published quarterly by Elsevier Inc., 360 Park Avenue South, New York, NY 10010-1710. Months of issue are January, April, July, and October. Business and Editorial Offices: 1600 John F. Kennedy Blvd., Suite 1800, Philadelphia, PA 19103-2899. Periodicals postage paid at New York, NY and additional mailing offices. Subscription prices are $548.00 per year for US individuals, $1234.00 per year for US institutions, $100.00 per year for US students and residents, $613.00 per year for Canadian individuals, $1,259.00 per year for Canadian institutions, $682.00 per year for international individuals, $1,259.00 per year for international institutions, $100.00 per year for Canadian and $305.00 per year for international students/residents. To receive student/resident rate, orders must be accompanied by name of affiliated institution, date of term, and the *signature* of program/residency coordinator on institution letterhead. Orders will be billed at individual rate until proof of status is received. Foreign air speed delivery is included in all *Clinics* subscription prices. All prices are subject to change without notice. **POSTMASTER:** Send address changes to *Clinics in Plastic Surgery*, Elsevier Health Sciences Division, Subscription Customer Service, 3251 Riverport Lane, Maryland Heights, MO 63043. **Customer Service: 1-800-654-2452 (US and Canada). From outside of the United States and Canada, call 314-447-8871. Fax: 314-447-8029. E-mail: JournalsCustomerService-usa@elsevier.com (for print support); JournalsOnline-Support-usa@elsevier.com (for online support).**

Reprints. For copies of 100 or more of articles in this publication, please contact the Commercial Reprints Department, Elsevier Inc., 360 Park Avenue South, New York, New York 10010-1710. Tel.: +1-212-633-3874; Fax: +1-212-633-3820; E-mail: reprints@elsevier.com.

Clinics in Plastic Surgery is covered in *Current Contents, EMBASE/Excerpta Medica, Science Citation Index, MEDLINE/ PubMed (Index Medicus), ASCA, and ISI/BIOMED.*

Contributors

EDITORS

DOUGLAS S. STEINBRECH, MD, FACS
Alpha Male Plastic Surgery, New York, Los
Angeles, Chicago, Gotham Plastic Surgery,
Owner, New York, New York, USA

ALAN MATARASSO, MD, FACS
Clinical Professor of Surgery, Hofstra
University/Northwell School of Medicine,
Manhattan Eye, Ear and Throat Hospital,
Lenox Hill Hospital, New York, New York,
USA

AUTHORS

FRANCISCO G. BRAVO, MD, PhD
Private Practice, Clinica Gomez Bravo, Madrid,
Spain

PAUL N. CHUGAY, MD, FACS
Private Practice - Chugay Cosmetic Surgery,
Long Beach, California, USA

ARMANDO A. DAVILA, BS, MD
Hurwitz Center for Plastic Surgery, Adjunct
Assistant Professor of Plastic Surgery, UNLV
School of Medicine, Las Vegas, Nevada, USA

DINO ELYASSNIA, MD
Marten Clinic of Plastic Surgery,
San Francisco, California, USA

DENNIS J. HURWITZ, BS, MD, FACS
Clinical Professor of Plastic Surgery, President
of the Hurwitz Center for Plastic Surgery,
University of Pittsburgh Medical School,
Pittsburgh, Pennsylvania, USA

TIMOTHY MARTEN, MD
Marten Clinic of Plastic Surgery,
San Francisco, California, USA

ALAN MATARASSO, MD, FACS
Clinical Professor of Surgery, Hofstra
University/Northwell School of Medicine,
Manhattan Eye, Ear and Throat Hospital, Lenox
Hill Hospital, New York, New York, USA

VINAY RAO, MD, MPH
Division of Plastic Surgery, The Warren Alpert
Medical School of Brown University,
Providence, Rhode Island, USA

DARREN M. SMITH, MD, FACS
Private Practice, New York, New York, USA

MICHAEL J. STEIN, MD, FRCSC
Manhattan Eye, Ear and Throat Hospital,
Lenox Hill Hospital, New York, New York,
USA

DAVID M. STRAUGHAN, MD
Division of Plastic and Reconstructive Surgery,
Massachusetts General Hospital, Boston,
Massachusetts, USA

PATRICK K. SULLIVAN, MD
The Warren Alpert Medical School of Brown
University, Providence, Rhode Island, USA

RICHARD J. WARREN, MD, FRCSC
Clinical Professor of Surgery, University of
British Columbia, Vancouver, British Columbia,
Canada

MICHAEL J. YAREMCHUK, MD
Division of Plastic and Reconstructive Surgery,
Massachusetts General Hospital, Boston,
Massachusetts, USA

Contents

> The upper lid-brow junction is a complex anatomic zone that undergoes many interconnected age-related changes. Although considerable effort has gone into defining the ideal female eye and brow, no such work has been done for the male. Typically, men develop forehead and glabellar lines in conjunction with either upper lid hooding, brow ptosis, or blepharoptosis, whereas some men develop hollowing of the upper lid sulcus. Physical examination defines which features predominate. Treatment can be nonsurgical or surgical. The surgical options include upper lid blepharoplasty, various types of brow lifting or brow shaping, ptosis repair, and fat grafting.

> Periorbital changes in men occur similarly to in women and may result in a need for correction through blepharoplasty. Lower lid techniques vary, but the authors prefer a transconjunctival approach that may extend into a retroseptal approach in men. Using this approach, excess fat can be excised and even redraped with orbitomalar retaining ligament release. Optimal outcomes are achieved when the surgical technique is targeted to correct the palpebromalar and nasojugal grooves, which are often the main concern for patients presenting to the office. Lower lid stabilization, support/tightening procedures are critical to prevent lower lid malposition and to ensure complete restoration of a youthful lower lid contour.

> Surgeons operating on the male face now understand that male facial aesthetics differ from those in women and that attractive masculinity is not as closely correlated with youth and beauty as is femininity. Men generally seek a somewhat different outcome from facial rejuvenation surgery, which has led to a rethinking of techniques that have evolved mainly to treat facial aging in women. Modified techniques have emerged and more refined and appropriate aesthetic goals have subsequently been sought that allow rejuvenation and improvement of the male face while preserving a natural, masculine appearance free of signs that surgery has been performed.

Specialists seeking successful outcomes in male facial rejuvenation must be able to achieve optimal definition in the neck and submental region in order provide their patients with balanced and natural results. A thorough understanding of male jawline and neck surface aesthetics is described and its relevance to perceived age, attractiveness, and body mass index is presented. The neck lift technique described is based on the pursuit of 2 distinct objectives managed independently: (1) Volume contouring or reduction, which is mainly accomplished in the deep structures of the neck beneath the platysma and (2) superficial redraping, which consists of the management of the platysma itself and of the overlying subcutaneous fat and skin. A dual-plane approach to the neck is used, meaning 2 different dissection planes are carried out. In the area cranial to the submandibular-cervical junction line (ie, submandibular segment), a plane is developed both superficial and deep to the platysma, while in the area caudal to this line (ie, cervical segment), dissection is carried out only deep to the platysma, leaving the muscle attached to its overlying skin. A description of the technique is presented as well as its complications and indications for surgical neck enhancement.

 Video content accompanies this article at http://www.plasticsurgery.theclinics.com.

The size and shape of the chin and mandible are fundamental to sexual dimorphism. Deficiencies in these structures distract from the male facial esthetic. When deficient, these areas of the facial skeleton can be augmented by alloplastic augmentation or skeletal rearrangement. This article discusses these alternatives with emphasis on the design and techniques of alloplastic skeletal augmentation.

Although body contouring has long been considered a female-dominated market, growing popularity among men has led to shifting market focus. The increase in male body contouring surgery has been fueled by increased recognition of its safety and efficacy, decreased stigma via social media awareness, and increasing desire among men seeking to remain competitive in the workforce. The growth of bariatric surgery has only compounded such trends, with a growing population of men seeking excisional procedures following massive weight loss. The authors review key features of the modern male abdominoplasty, with respect to anatomy, patient selection, surgical technique, and postoperative outcomes.

 Video content accompanies this article at http://www.plasticsurgery.theclinics.com.

Contemporary management of gynecomastia includes transareolar excision of gland, disruption of inframammary fold, ultrasonic-assisted lipoplasty with muscular definition, bipolar radiofrequency tightening, pedicled NAC mastopexy with boomerang pattern excision and J torsoplasty, NAC grafts with hockey stick excision pattern, and pectoralis muscle lipoaugmentation. Therapeutic options are arranged across a modified Simon classification. The aesthetic goal is near total glandular reduction, with proper position and shape of the nipple areolar complexes, and masculinity with skin adherence reflecting musculoskeleton. Clinical cases demonstrate these multiple approaches, successes, and pitfalls. Complications relate to delayed healing caused by excessive closure tension or inadequate or inappropriate treatment.

High-Definition Liposuction in Men

Michael J. Stein and Alan Matarasso

Liposuction is the most common procedure in plastic surgery and becoming increasingly common in male patients. Recently, liposuction has evolved from a procedure whose goal was primarily fat extraction, to one that sculpts tissue with the goal of enhancing muscular definition. The popularity of high-definition liposuction has increased rapidly due to visibility on social media and has broadened the patient population presenting for liposuction, particularly among men. Herein, the authors review patient selection, surgical technique, and postoperative outcomes following high-definition liposuction in male patients.

Calf Augmentation

Paul N. Chugay

Calf augmentation is a very gratifying procedure with immediate and reproducible results. The procedure can be successfully performed by novice and expert surgeons alike, making sure to respect anatomic boundaries and avoiding over dissection. Major complications can be avoided with meticulous closure of the wound and restriction of activity postoperatively as well as use of compression stockings until sufficient scar tissue has developed.

The Role of Energy-Based Devices in Male Body Contouring

Darren M. Smith

Energy-based devices extend the indications of traditional procedures in male body contouring. Devices currently available in this space may be noninvasive or minimally invasive. These devices use heat to destroy fat or tighten soft tissue and electromagnetic energy to build muscle mass. Thoughtful deployment of these technologies in isolation or in combination with each other or more traditional approaches can improve outcomes in male body contouring without an increase in scar burden. Patient selection and education are essential in maximizing satisfaction with these procedures.

CLINICS IN PLASTIC SURGERY

ISSUE OF RELATED INTEREST

Facial Plastic Surgery Clinics
https://www.facialplastic.theclinics.com/
Otolaryngologic Clinics
https://www.oto.theclinics.com/

THE CLINICS ARE AVAILABLE ONLINE!
Access your subscription at:
www.theclinics.com

Preface
Male Plastic Surgery: The Current State-of-the-Art

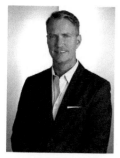

Douglas S. Steinbrech, MD, FACS
Editor

Back in 2004, when I finished my Plastic Surgery Residency at the NYU and started my practice, I really had felt that I was fortunate enough to have had excellent training in Aesthetic Plastic Surgery. With the esteemed professors at NYU, and particularly Manhattan Eye and Ear Attendings that taught us so many of the greatest techniques in Aesthetic Plastic Surgery, I thought I was quite prepared to operate—on women.

Yes, something was lacking. Although the halls of the OR were lined with some of the world's greatest icons in Aesthetic Plastic Surgery, by far, the majority of the procedures were performed on women. And in the MEETH Resident clinics, by far, the majority of patients seen were women.

Why was this? This was because, in general, techniques specific to men were not taught in our residencies, and we as surgeons lacked the training, skills, and practice to gain confidence to provide consistent results we were proud of for our staff, our patients, our residents, and ourselves. In fact, we as a medical community went as far as to vilify many male patients as "S.I.M.O.N.s", and that our residents and staff should be aware and avoid these. Since then, it has been my observations that men make excellent patients just like women.

After I started my own private practice, I immediately had many male friends who had been waiting to have aesthetic plastic surgery procedures, but I noticed that there was not a lot of information out there. During that period of time, with the legendary Sherrell J. Aston, and the meteorically rising Dr Jennifer Walden, we set out to construct an 864-page textbook about Plastic Surgery: *Aesthetic Plastic Surgery*, which was primarily aimed at women. But when it was time to put together a second edition, I was approached about another textbook, specifically for Male Aesthetic Plastic Surgery.

Also, during this time, we were noticing a rise in the numbers of men in my practice. With this in mind, we set out to establish The New York Institute of Male Plastic Surgery to develop techniques, to educate residents and practicing Plastic Surgeons, and to study safely tested devices to allow interested Plastic Surgeons to be able to learn these techniques, grow their practices, and provide more services geared to men.

So, why the need for this supplement on men? Over the past 2 decades, the authors in this issue have continued to work on improving and developing these techniques to be able to provide the best results in their thriving practices. All at the same time, dramatic improvements in lipocell transfer and technologies, such as alloplastic augmentation, have taken place.

Clin Plastic Surg 49 (2022) ix–x
https://doi.org/10.1016/j.cps.2022.02.004
0094-1298/22/© 2022 Published by Elsevier Inc.

We feel like this is just the beginning of a great journey, and we hope that this supplement will inspire many readers to continue to grow in attracting men to be able to provide excellent treatment and results for them. We feel that this is indeed the golden era of the growth of Men's Plastic Surgery and hope that many surgeons will continue.

I wish you the same great interest in this area that I have felt and great success in developing your armamentarium to include more male-based procedures for your patients and your practice.

After all, 51% of the world population is men.

Douglas S. Steinbrech, MD, FACS
Alpha Male Plastic Surgery
New York, Los Angeles, Chicago

Gotham Plastic Surgery
60 East 56th Street, Suite 302
New York, NY 10022, USA

E-mail address:
dss@drsteinbrech.com

Preface
Plastic Surgery in Men

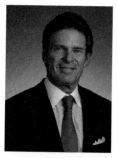

Alan Matarasso, MD, FACS
Editor

Historically, when reviewing the aesthetic literature, men did not represent a distinct entity; they were infrequently written about and actually more often an afterthought. Techniques devoted exclusively to men were rarely described. Rather, procedures used in the preponderance of our female patients were adapted to men, all while knowing the special challenges and often higher complication rates that men exhibit. Over the last few decades, patients and society inevitably changed and evolved; cultural norms and morals shifted, and a notable rise in men seeking cosmetic enhancement ensued.

Indeed, this has been accelerated by the ubiquitous social media and general consumer-viewed content, featuring men demonstrating greater acceptance and larger numbers.

In parallel to the mainstream acceptance of male plastic surgery has been a development in procedures based on their unique anatomical features and goals. The need for specific techniques evolved to the point that we now recognize and develop operations designed exclusively for men. Although many techniques in women and men may be different, there are procedural and conceptual similarities as well, such as the "daddy do over" and its parallel, the "mommy makeover."

As physicians adapt to the requirements necessary for successful male outcomes and society adapts to this phenomenon, the population will continue to age, and the demands for male plastic surgery are expected to continue to rise.

The fact that an issue of *Clinics in Plastic Surgery* is devoted exclusively to an entire segment of individuals is a testimony to the importance of education on this topic. The authors assembled herein have lent their time and given great efforts to go beyond the demands of daily practice and share their hard-earned expertise with colleagues interested in this topic. Thank you! We hope that this issue improves our knowledge and our patients' experiences and outcomes and inspires further advances in this field.

Alan Matarasso, MD, FACS
Hofstra University/
Northwell School of Medicine
1009 Park Avenue
New York, NY 10028, USA

E-mail address:
amatarasso@drmatarasso.com

Clin Plastic Surg 49 (2022) xi
https://doi.org/10.1016/j.cps.2022.02.002
0094-1298/22/© 2022 Published by Elsevier Inc.

Upper Blepharoplasty and Brow Rejuvenation in Men

Richard J. Warren, MD, FRCSC

KEYWORDS

• Eyebrow • Frown lines • Blepharoplasty • Brow lift • Ptosis • Fat graft

KEY POINTS

- The ideal male upper lid brow junction is different than in the female. Surgical objectives in the male should also be different.
- Men have lower eyebrows. As upper eyelid hodding develops with age, this leads to chronic brow elevation.
- Rejuvenation surgery in the male frequently benefits from a combined procedure to stabilize eyebrow poisition, while reducing upper eyelid hooding.
- Conservative treatment in males is a safe approach.

INTRODUCTION

The upper eyelid-brow junction is a complex anatomic zone that undergoes many interconnected changes as we age. Surgical procedures to rejuvenate this area are some of the most impactful operations in aesthetic surgery. However, ill-advised, or poorly designed surgery can result in suboptimal results that are difficult or impossible to correct.

The key to successful treatment of this area is knowledge of the anatomy and a sophisticated understanding of the way in which upper lids and foreheads age. Compared with the female upper eyelid-brow junction, there are significant differences in the male. This concept has been challenging for aesthetic surgeons because most patients are women, and surgical literature has focused on the aesthetic ideals of the female eye. Furthermore, the aesthetic goals of men are usually more limited. Simply put, most men presenting for rejuvenation of the periorbital area want to look a little more like they did in their youth. They are usually not seeking a stylized male appearance and they do not want to be feminized.

AESTHETIC ISSUES—HISTORY AND BACKGROUND

Historically, humans have enhanced the periorbital area using makeup, tattoos, eyebrow plucking, and piercing. As esthetic surgery developed, authors tried to define the esthetic objectives of brow lift and blepharoplasty procedures. Almost all this work focused on women.

The modern era can be traced to 1975, when Westmore, a make-up artist, suggested that for the ideal female eye, the lateral and medial ends of the brow should be at the same level and the brow should peak above the lateral limbus.[1] Gunter and Antabus advanced this concept by assessing female models (**Fig. 1**). They introduced the concept of the eye at the center of an oval that measured equidistant from pupil to the eyebrow above and to the nasojugal groove below[2,3] (**Fig. 2**). Some authors have tried to define female attractiveness using the Golden Proportion, the seemingly attractive ratio of 1 to 1.618[4,5] (**Fig. 3**).

The normal male eyebrow is typically described as lower than the female, less arched, and horizontally positioned along the supraorbital rim.[2,4,6] In normal men, deep set eyes are associated with

There are no funding sources for the author of this article.
University of British Columbia and Vancouver Plastic Surgery Center, 777 West Broadway, Suite 1000, Vancouver, British Columbia V5Z4J7, Canada
E-mail address: richardwarren@shaw.ca

Clin Plastic Surg 49 (2022) 197–212
https://doi.org/10.1016/j.cps.2021.12.006
0094-1298/22/© 2022 Elsevier Inc. All rights reserved.

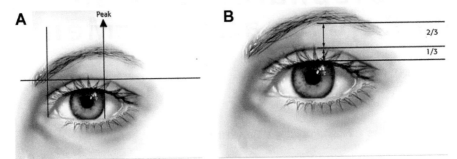

Fig. 1. (*A*) According to Gunter and Antabus, in the attractive female eye, the lateral eyebrow is higher than the medial with a gentle peak lateral to the iris. (*B*) The ratio of visible eyelid skin (pretarsal show) is approximately one-third and at most one-half the distance from the lash line to the lower border of the eyebrow. (*Courtesy* Doug Peters / Alamy Stock Photo, WENN Rights Ltd / Alamy Stock Photo and Retro AdArchives / Alamy Stock Photo.)

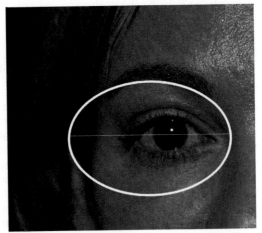

Fig. 2. For the attractive female eye, the oval theory holds that an oval formed by the eyebrow above and the nasojugal groove below should have the pupil at its equator.

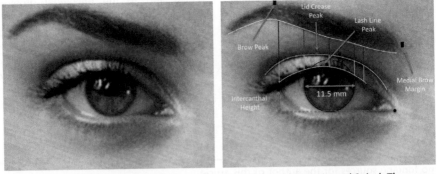

Fig. 3. A modern version of the attractive female eye based on the Golden Ratio and Spiral. The upper eyelid fold to tarsal show ratio ranges from 1.8 to 3.0 with the greatest tarsal show located laterally. The lateral lid crease peaks lateral to the pupil and the brow peaks lateral to that. (*From* Vaca EE, Bricker JT, Helenowski I, Park ED, Alghoul MS. Identifying Aesthetically Appealing Upper Eyelid Topographic Proportions. Aesthet Surg J. 2019 Jul 12;39(8):824-834; with permission.)

lower eyebrow position, whereas more prominent eyes have a higher eyebrow position.[6] To date, there has been no scientific literature looking at the "ideal" parameters that would define attractiveness in a man.

To address the question of male attractiveness, **Fig. 4** shows 3 men, considered to be the leading male models in the world at the time of this writing.[7] For the purpose of this discussion, it is assumed that these are attractive men. Compared with the well-studied female ideal, there are obvious differences. With a combination of low eyebrows and a full upper sulcus, the upper lid-brow junction is a very crowded space in these men.

DISCUSSION—AGING CHANGES IN THE MALE FOREHEAD

The most obvious age-related changes in the male forehead are skin furrows caused by muscle contraction. Men have thicker forehead skin than women, which results in deeper lines once they have formed. This has therapeutic implications because deep forehead lines in thick male skin are less likely to be eradicated. Fortunately, older males often prefer the more mature appearance caused, in part by lines on the forehead.

Glabellar frown lines are caused by the contraction of corrugator supercilii, depressor supercilii, and the procerus muscles, all of which depress the medial brow (**Fig. 5**). Transverse forehead lines are caused by frontalis contraction in an unconscious effort to clear the obstruction to visual fields. The most common cause of visual field impairment is upper eyelid hooding. Other potential etiologies are blepharoptosis and an intrinsic drop in eyebrow level—something that occurs in approximately one-third of men and women.[8] Any of these issues will affect the line of sight. Because male eyebrows tend to be low and the upper lid skin fold often rests on the eyelashes, there is not much margin for change. Therefore, as they age, most men develop compensatory tone in their frontalis, resulting in transverse forehead lines (**Fig. 6**).

DISCUSSION—AGING CHANGES IN THE MALE UPPER EYELID
Upper Lid Soft Tissue

By design, upper eyelid skin is redundant, allowing for proper eye closure and protection of the globe. The upper eyelid fold is the curtain of skin, with or without redundant orbicularis, that creates upper lid hooding. The upper lid crease is the curved line where pretarsal skin meets preseptal skin.

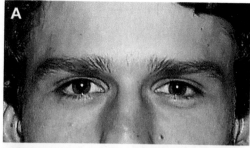
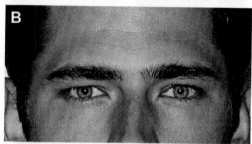
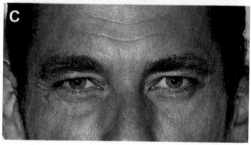

Fig. 4. The top three male models in the world in 2019 are shown. In all three men, the eyebrows are low and flat. The medial end of the eyebrow begins at or medial to the medial canthus. The eyebrow hair pattern is naturally full. In the two younger men (A and B), the eyebrows are thicker medially and in the older man (C), they are thicker laterally which gives the illusion of a lateral arch. Visibility of the upper lids (tarsal show) is minimal, especially in the mid pupillary line where the eyelid fold rests directly on the eyelashes in two of the models. In the older model (C), the upper lid skin fold rests on the eyelashes across the entire eyelid. In all 3 models, the upper lid sulcus is crowded with the distance from mid pupil to lower eyebrow border estimated to be less than 10 mm. (*Modified from* GQ Staff. These are the 10 Richest Male Models in the World. February 26, 2019. https://www.gq.com.au/success/finance/these-are-the-10-richest-male-models-in-the-world/image-gallery/88fc80680016ae7933d4ad7d9f2c3de1?pos=3.)

The crease is tethered to the levator aponeurosis and can be found at different levels—lower in Asians. The area between the eyebrows and the upper lids is the upper lid sulcus. The amount of visible pretarsal skin (tarsal show) is determined by the level of the crease and the magnitude of the skin fold. With age, the upper lid skin fold usually becomes more redundant and less elastic,

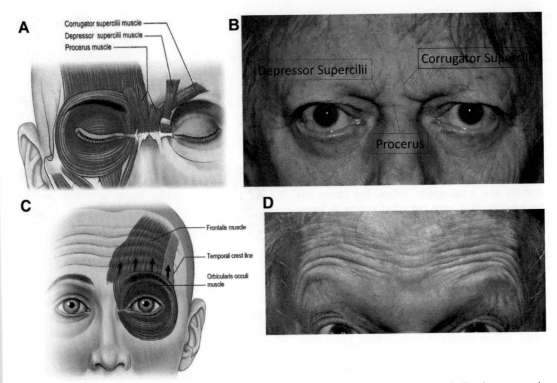

Fig. 5. (*A*) The glabellar frown muscles. (*B*) The furrow lines caused by chronic action of glabellar frown muscles. (*C*) The frontalis muscle is the only brow elevator. Its action is strongest centrally and weakest laterally. (*D*) The furrows caused by frontalis. (*From* [*A, B*] Warren R. Chapter 23: Non-Endoscopic Limited Incision Browlift. In: Aston SJ, Steinbrech D, and Walden J, eds. Aesthetic Plastic Surgery. Saunders Elsevier; 2009: 263-274. [*C*] Warren RJ. Chapter 7: Forehead rejuvenation. In: Rubin PJ, Neligan P, eds. Plastic Surgery: Volume 2: Aesthetic Surgery. 4th ed. Elsevier: 2018;273—287.e2.)

leading to a soft tissue curtain that hangs down, hiding the pretarsal skin as seen in **Fig. 7**.

Directly under the skin and contributing to soft tissue volume is the orbicularis oculi with its 3 components: pretarsal, preseptal, and orbital. It is the preseptal muscle that contributes to upper lid hooding (**Fig. 8**). In the aging male, retroseptal fat may become protuberant, leading to excess soft tissue fullness. The retro-orbicularis oculi fat (ROOF) adds fullness to the supralateral orbital rim. Occasionally, a ptotic lacrimal gland contributes to lateral lid fullness.

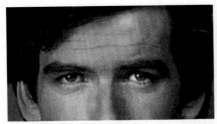
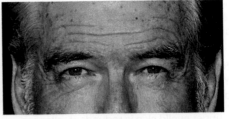

Fig. 6. In youth, this man had the eyebrow configuration of an attractive male: low and transverse. The upper lid skin fold rests on the lashes with no tarsal show centrally but slight tarsal show laterally. With age, as the upper lid skin fold becomes more redundant, he subconsciously contracts the frontalis muscle, lifting the eyebrows to clear his line of sight. The eyebrows are now higher than they were in his youth. Laterally, where the frontalis action is less, the brow is slightly lower, and the upper lid skin fold completely hides the pretarsal skin. (*Courtesy* PictureLux / The Hollywood Archive / Alamy Stock Photo and UPI / Alamy Stock Photo.)

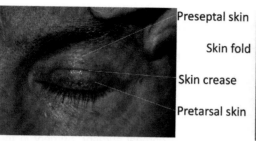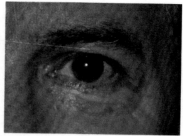

Preseptal skin

Skin fold

Skin crease

Pretarsal skin

Fig. 7. Terminology for upper lid skin crease and fold.

Alternatively, some aging males appear to lose volume in the upper lid sulcus, and with it, the youthful fullness normally seen at the upper lid junction. A key factor in this process is the gradual enlargement of the bony orbit.[9] Combined with the effect of gravity in the upright position, fat may bulge in the lower lid, and appear to be lost in the upper lids, as in **Fig. 9**A. Some patients may present with what appears to be premature aging due to aggressive fat removal during blepharoplasty as seen in **Fig. 9**B. In all cases of upper sulcus hollowing, soft tissue augmentation is the appropriate treatment; tissue excision will not correct the problem.

Eyelid Ptosis

In men and women, the upper lid normally covers the top 2 mm of the iris. If more of the iris is covered, the eyelids look ptotic.[2] One study in England found blepharoptosis in 11.5% of patients over age 50 years, whereas a study in Korea found an incidence of 32% over age 70 years.[10,11] The clinical implication is that in the age group of patients who present for blepharoplasty, many will have senile ptosis. This condition is caused by

thinning and stretching of the levator aponeurosis as seen in **Fig. 10**A. The result is a recognizable triad of a hollow upper lid sulcus, increased tarsal show, and eyebrow elevation as seen in **Fig. 10**B. In the presence of ptosis, a return to the appearance of youth cannot be achieved unless the underlying ptosis problem is corrected.

CLINICAL PRESENTATION

When a man presents for rejuvenation of the upper lid-brow junction, there may be aesthetic concerns, functional concerns, or both. Functional concerns typically relate to an obstruction of vision caused by eyelid ptosis, eyebrow ptosis, or upper lid dermatochalasis—alone or in combination. If this is the presenting issue, care must be taken to document the level of the eyelids, the function of the levator and to do visual field testing.

In the aesthetic realm, the typical concerns of men are upper lid hooding, glabellar frown lines, and transverse forehead lines. Some men may have tried neurotoxin injections but are disenchanted with the repeated visits required; they are looking for permanence.

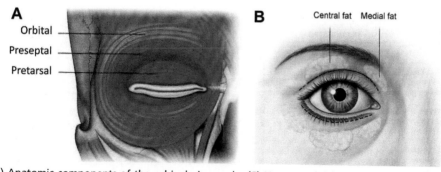

Fig. 8. (*A*) Anatomic components of the orbicularis muscle. (*B*) Upper eyelid fat compartments. ([A] *From* Jelks GW, Jelks EB, Chiu ES, and Steinbrech DS. Chapter 10: Secondary blepharoplasty: Techniques. In: Rubin PJ, Neligan P, eds. Plastic Surgery: Volume 2: Aesthetic Surgery. 4th ed. Elsevier: 326-349.e2. [B] *Adapted from* Saadeh P. Chapter 29: Conventional Upper and Lower Blepharoplasty. In: Aston SJ, Steinbrech D, and Walden J, eds. Aesthetic Plastic Surgery. Saunders Elsevier; 2009:321-328.)

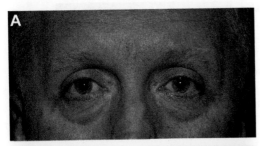

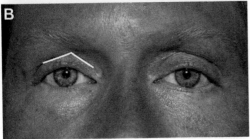

Fig. 9. (*A*) A 53-year-old man with age-related hollowing of the upper lid sulcus. The orbit has enlarged. With the effect of gravity and the loss of support in the lower lid septum, orbital fat bulges forward in the lower half of the orbit and recedes in the upper half. (*B*) This man has an A-frame deformity in the upper lid sulcus. This was caused by overly aggressive fat removal during upper lid blepharoplasty.

It is rare for a man to present with a concern about hollowing in his upper lid sulcus. Unless this has been pointed out previously, most men first learn about this issue during their consultation.

Uncommonly, an aesthetically astute male may have specific requests that reference an ideal male appearance. Such an individual may demonstrate his objectives with photographs of celebrities and models. A frank discussion regarding

realistic expectations is critical with these individuals.

PATIENT HISTORY

Before aesthetic eyelid surgery, medical topics that should be addressed are thyroid disease, true blepharochalasis with a history of recurrent eyelid edema, dry eye syndrome, and a history of recent corneal surgery. Surgery in the presence of these conditions can still be safe if appropriate measures are taken. When in doubt, preoperative ophthalmologic consultation is recommended.

It is important to know if the patient has had nonsurgical treatments in the past, including neurotoxin injections, soft tissue filler injections, or skin resurfacing procedures around the eye. A proper assessment of the forehead requires that no active neurotoxin be present.

With aging, it is normal for patients to forget what they used to look like. Old photographs, preferably nonsmiling, are especially useful in this regard. Images from a man's youth will also prompt him to reflect on whether he really liked his eyes the way they were or if he would like a fundamental change.

PHYSICAL EXAMINATION OF THE UPPER LID/ BROW JUNCTION

For proper assessment, the patient should be positioned vertically. In the supine position, gravity is neutralized, and the eyebrows will migrate upward. Also, when supine, orbital fat sinks into the orbit, changing the soft tissue variables in the upper lid sulcus.

The rest of the face should be assessed, especially the lower lid cheek junction, which aesthetically balances the upper lid-brow junction on the esthetic oval principle.[2,4] Some asymmetries in

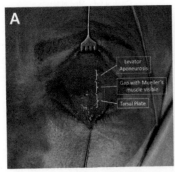

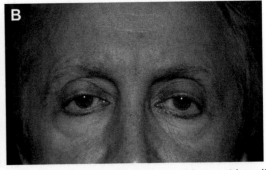

Fig. 10. (*A*) The clinical findings of senile ptosis during blepharoplasty. (*B*) A 50-year-old man with eyelid ptosis. In response to levator aponeurosis dehiscence from the tarsal plate, the levator muscle retracts. This pulls the pretarsal skin and retroseptal fat superiorly and posteriorly toward Whitnall's ligament. The result is a hollow upper lid sulcus with increased tarsal show and compensatory eyebrow elevation.

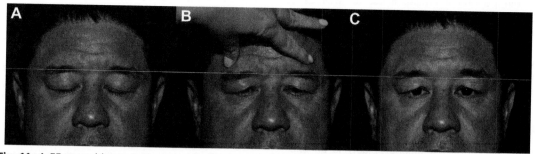

Fig. 11. A 55-year-old man is shown with chronic eyebrow elevation in response to upper eyelid hooding. (*A*) Relaxed with eyes closed. (*B*) Attempted forward gaze with eyebrows held in a relaxed position. (*C*) Normal forward gaze with eyebrows lifted. This man's eyebrows do not have a stable position. If an upper blepharoplasty is done, the resting eyebrow level will drop.

the face are to be expected, especially in the periorbital area where brow height and shape are commonly asymmetric.

Focusing on the forehead and eyebrows, the nature of the forehead skin, the hairline, the depth of furrows, and the strength of frown musculature is assessed. Eyebrow shape and height is noted and the stability of eyebrow position is assessed, as in **Fig. 11.**

In the upper lid sulcus, the amount of soft tissue is estimated. Often the only bulging fat of concern is a small pocket medially. If lateral fullness is present, ROOF and the lacrimal gland should be assessed. Soft tissue hooding can be determined using nontoothed forceps to estimate skin excess. The level of the natural eyelid creases is noted.

The eyelid level should be determined. To determine the function of Mueller's muscle, a drop of phenylephrine can be placed into the eye. With this test, a normal Mueller's muscle will lift the edge of the upper lid by around 2 mm.[12]

If ptosis surgery is contemplated, levator function should be documented. This is done by asking the patient to look down at the floor and then look up to the ceiling and record the distance moved by the upper lid margin. Normal is 12 mm or above. When levator function is good, in the setting of senile acquired ptosis, the patient is a candidate for plication of the levator aponeurosis during blepharoplasty. Frequently, senile ptosis is bilateral but masked by Hering's law of equal innervation.[13]

Plastic surgeons can easily examine the anterior segment of the eye with a simple light, looking for anything abnormal, including cataracts. The meibomian glands can be assessed by gently massaging the eyelid margins looking for discharge. If there is discharge, a diagnosis of meibomianitis is possible. This may require an oral antibiotic in the postoperative period if blepharoplasty is done.

TREATMENT OBJECTIVES

It is during the consultation that important decisions are made, and a treatment plan is formulated. After physical examination, the patient's concerns must be correlated with the surgeon's anatomic findings. In practical terms, a mirror can be misleading because of the tendency for people to raise their eyebrows when looking at a reflection of themselves. Computer imaging can help, although personally, I use a life-sized printed photograph on which I can draw my plans and demonstrate what I think the changes will likely be.

Frequently, what the patient feels is a simple problem is multifactorial. To understand these issues, men appreciate seeing photographs of other men with similar anatomy, along with photographic results of their surgery.

NONSURGICAL PROCEDURES

No discussion about Brow Rejuvenation would be complete without some mention of nonsurgical therapies, although the focus of this article is on surgery.

For many men, the first concern with their aging face is the development of frown lines in the glabellar region as seen earlier in **Fig. 5.** Botulinum toxin injection is an excellent first choice to deal with lines caused by the corrugator supercilii, the depressor supercilii, and the procerus.[14] The frontalis is also amenable to treatment, although the potential for a lower brow position or altered brow shape must be taken into consideration.

With skillful use of neurotoxin, the elevator and depressors of the eyebrow can be targeted together, allowing subtle changes to be made in the shape of the eyebrow.[15]

There are a host of soft tissue fillers available, and this topic is beyond the range of this article. However, the appropriate filler can be used to smooth periorbital crease lines, as well as to augment volume around the orbital rim and within the upper lid sulcus.[15–17]

Skin resurfacing has shown its usefulness for eyelid skin as well as the forehead. Chemical peels, laser resurfacing and dermabrasion can all be used in the appropriate clinical setting.[15]

UPPER LID BLEPHAROPLASTY

Classically, upper lid blepharoplasty is an excisional procedure. The indications are soft tissue hooding with or without bulging orbital fat. The surgical objective depends on the patient's goals and anatomic findings—all balanced by our knowledge that the ideal male anatomy is one with minimal tarsal show and a significant amount of upper sulcus fullness.

Surgical markings are done preoperatively in the upright position, as I prefer, or as others do, in the operating room with the patient supine. **Fig. 12** shows a patient being marked in the upright position. In almost all men, it is necessary to extend the lateral marking past the lateral canthus to account for lateral hooding.

The surgery can be done under local anesthetic with or without sedation. The skin is removed first and, in many cases, that is the only excision required (**Fig. 13**). The routine removal of

orbicularis was once common, but it is now understood that soft tissue bulk provided by muscle is a youthful feature and an attractive component in men.[18] However, the asymmetric removal of muscle can be useful to address asymmetries in balancing the soft tissue bulk that will remain after soft tissue excision. Also, if the eyebrows are low, but a patient does not want brow lift surgery, the removal of some muscle bulk may be necessary to adequately remove enough soft tissue, especially laterally. The configuration of the orbit influences this decision, depending on the openness of the upper lid sulcus and the level of the eyebrow. High supraorbital rims with prominent globes call for more conservative skin removal, whereas low-lying orbital rims with deep set eyes lend themselves to more extensive skin removal.

The orbicularis muscle is incised to gain access for fat removal, to reposition the lacrimal gland, or for ptosis repair. Although the medial fat compartment often causes a slight bulge that requires treatment, care must be taken not to over-resect restroseptal fat, especially centrally, creating a hollow upper sulcus as in **Fig. 9**A.

During an upper blepharoplasty, frown musculature can be attenuated through direct transpalpebral resection (**Fig. 14**). This useful technique is done through an upper blepharoplasty approach to access the corrugator supercilli as well as the

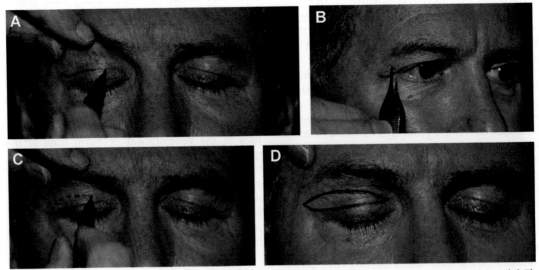

Fig. 12. Preoperative marking for an upper lid blepharoplasty with the patient in that upright position. (*A*) The natural lid crease is marked with the patient's eyes closed. Laterally, the incision turns slightly upward into a crow's foot wrinkle superior to the lateral canthus. Medially, there is slight upturn without extending onto the nose. (*B*) With the brow released, forceps are used to estimate hooding and marks are made. (*C*) The orientation marks are joined to complete marking of the planned skin removal. (*D*). The completed marking is fusiform in shape, usually widest laterally, with the upper and lower limbs of the marking roughly equal in length.

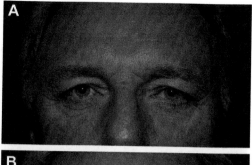

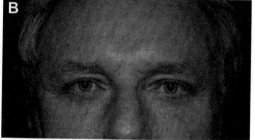

Fig. 13. (*A*) A 58-year-old man with upper lid hooding and stable eyebrow position. (*B*) 6 months after a skin only upper lid blepharoplasty.

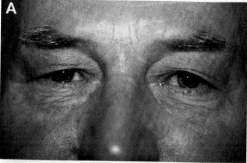

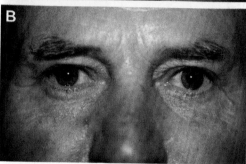

Fig. 15. Blepharoplasty in the setting of chronic brow elevation. (*A*) A 68-year-old man is shown with upper eyelid hooding and chronic frontalis contraction holding his eyebrows in an elevated position. (*B*) After upper lid blepharoplasty, the frontalis has relaxed and the eyebrows settle to a lower level. Patients must be forewarned of this possibility. To prevent the eyebrow level from dropping, a simultaneous brow stabilizing procedure is necessary.

depressor supercilii and the procerus muscles. When brow lift surgey is not being done, this method provides an alternative strategy to surgically attenuate frowning.[19]

A common side effect of upper lid blepharoplasty is postoperative relaxation of frontalis tone and a drop in eyebrow level. If this is not explained ahead of time, the patient may conclude that the blepharoplasty has "pulled" the eyebrows down. In **Fig. 15**, a patient with chronic brow elevation to compensate for upper lid hooding is shown before and after excisional blepharoplasty with the resulting drop in eyebrow position.

BROW LIFT

In recent times, there has been a decrease in the number of brow lift procedures being done, likely a result of injectable neurotoxins.[20] However, the variety of surgical options for brow lifting continues

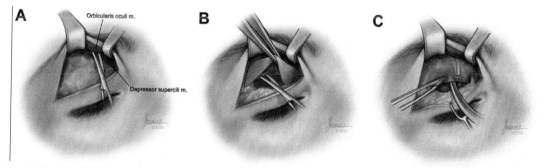

Fig. 14. Transpalpebral corrugator resection. (*A*) Through an open blepharoplasty incision, the orbicularis muscle is incised, and dissection proceeds superiorly in the plane between the orbicularis muscle and the orbital septum. (*B*) The depressor supercilii is being elevated here and overlies the darker colored and more friable corrugator. (*C*) Medially, a branch of the supratrochlear nerve pierces the corrugator. It is dissected, and the corrugator is removed lateral to that. When the volume of muscle is significant, a small fat graft is inserted. (*From* Guyuron B, Son JH. Transpalpebral Corrugator Resection: 25-Year Experience, Refinements and Additional Indications. Aesthetic Plast Surg. 2017 Apr;41(2):339-345; with permission.)

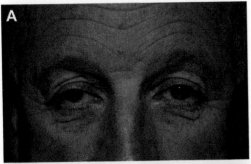

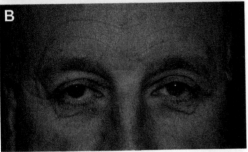

Fig. 16. Blepharoplasty with brow stabilization. (*A*) A 70-year-old man is shown with upper eyelid hooding and active frontalis contraction. (*B*) After upper lid blepharoplasty with removal of skin and a subcutaneous lateral brow lift, the brow position has been maintained.

to grow and many new techniques are well suited for men. Also, for many men, the prospect of a permanent or semipermanent result is more appealing than a long-term commitment to injections.

There are several aesthetic indications for brow lift surgery. The eyebrows can be lifted in whole or in part, thus changing either the overall height or the shape of the eyebrows. With some techniques, frown muscles can be removed. Elevating the eyebrows can clear an obstructed line of sight, resulting in relaxation of the frontalis and smoothing of transverse forehead lines. Lastly, in many patients with upper lid hooding who undergo blepharoplasty, a valid goal of brow lift surgery is not to lift the eyebrows, but rather, to stabilize brow position when the frontalis inevitably relaxes after blepharoplasty (**Fig. 16**).

The main clinical problem with most brow lift surgery is predictability and the likelihood of some relapse. Although upper lid blepharoplasty is accurate to the millimeter, brow lifting is not. This is particularly important in the male because the upper lid-brow junction can be a crowded space and a small drop in eyebrow level can have a significant effect on the upper lid sulcus.

Open Coronal Approach

The open coronal approach was long felt to be the gold standard against which other techniques

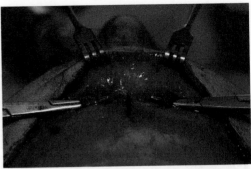

Fig. 17. An open coronal brow lift procedure. The wide surgical exposure allows for definitive soft tissue release, direct modification of frown musculature (corrugator muscles demonstrated here), and the opportunity for direct treatment of a prominent supraorbital ridge.

were measured. It still offers the advantages of complete surgical exposure, as seen in **Fig. 17**, good predictability and long-lasting results. The incision can be placed anywhere between the vertex and the anterior hairline, as seen in **Fig. 18**. The entire forehead is undermined, and orbital rim attachments can be released as necessary. Problems include the potential of permanently decreased scalp sensation and a long scar. In

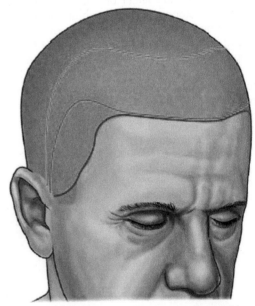

Fig. 18. Possible locations for an open coronal brow lift incision. Normally the incision is made full thickness, down to periosteum, 6 to 8 cms. behind anterior hairline. The flap is raised in the subgaleal plane. (*From* Warren RJ. Chapter 7: Forehead rejuvenation. In: Rubin PJ, Neligan P, eds. Plastic Surgery: Volume 2: Aesthetic Surgery. 4th ed. Elsevier; 2018;273-287.e2.)

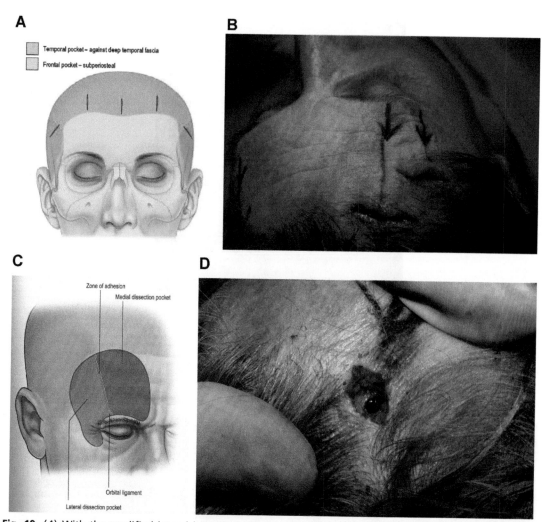

Fig. 19. (*A*) With the modified lateral brow technique, 5 dissection ports are used: central, paramedian, and lateral. The central port is eliminated if glabellar frown muscles are not being modified. (*B*) In balding men or men with thinning hair, the incisions can be made transverse, fitting into natural crease lines. (*C*) Through the paramedian and lateral ports, the lateral and medial dissection pockets are developed and then joined by dividing the zone of adhesion along the temporal crest line. Orbital rim galea attachments are divided medially past the supraorbital nerve and inferiorly past the lateral canthus—until clinically significant movement is achieved. (*D*) Three methods of fixation are used with the modified technique: suturing the superficial to the deep temporal fascia, bony fixation at the paramedian port (shown here), and suturing galea to galea through the lateral port. (*From* [*A*] Warren RJ. Chapter 7: Forehead rejuvenation. In: Rubin PJ, Neligan P, eds. Plastic Surgery: Volume 2: Aesthetic Surgery. 4th ed. Elsevier: 2018;273-287.e2. [*C*] Warren R. Chapter 23: Non-Endoscopic Limited Incision Browlift. In: Aston SJ, Steinbrech D, and Walden J, eds. Aesthetic Plastic Surgery. Saunders Elsevier; 2009: 263-274.)

men who have lost hair or may lose hair in the future, this scar is a significant deterrent. However, the open coronal brow lift is a powerful procedure and still has a place for men with a full head of hair and and heavy brow tissue.

Endoscopic Approach

The endoscopic approach accomplishes the same objectives as the open coronal, with the same deep dissection, but done through small nerve-sparing incisions.[21] It is well suited for the male patient because the small incisions can be used in a patient with thinning hair or no hair at all.[22] Problems with this technique are the training and specialized equipment required as well as predictability. Long-term studies show a range of results, with some relapse reported in most published series.[23,24] The reasons for failure are twofold. If the procedure fails in the early postoperative course, it is usually because of inadequate soft tissue

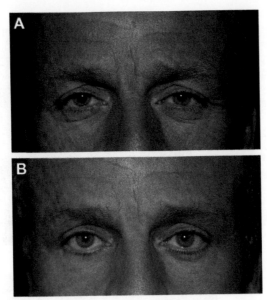

Fig. 20. (*A*) A 48-year-old man with periorbital brow ptosis and lower lid changes. (*B*) 12 months after modified lateral brow lift plus lower blepharoplasty and facelift.

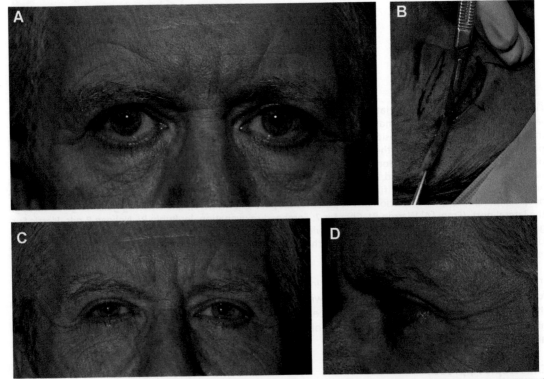

Fig. 21. A 50-year-old man who had a direct subcutaneous eyebrow lift in conjunction with blepharoplasty and lower lid canthopexy. (*A*) Preoperative brow ptosis and lower lid malposition. (*B*) Skin excision for direct brow lift. Hair follicles are protected and suturing is done with minimal tension. (*C*) Postoperative result at 1 year. (*D*) Direct brow lift scar at 1 year.

release around the orbital rim especially laterally. This is a technical problem that can be eliminated with experience. If it fails late, the problem is fixation. For that reason, a host of different fixation methods have been described.

For men with firm brow tissues where loose skin is not the defining problem, I use a 5 port endoscopic technique, as outlined in **Figs. 19 and 20**.[25] A postoperative bupivacaine block is used to help prevent postoperative headache and after 1 week, botulinum toxin is injected into the lateral orbicularis to help reduce the chances of recurrence.

Subcutaneous Approach

Subcutaneous techniques for brow lifting are well suited for many male patients who have deep transverse forehead lines or thick eyebrows—2 locations that disguise the necessary incisions. The eyebrow is a cutaneous structure, so in theory, repositioning the hair baring eyebrow skin is a logical approach. Incisions can be placed anywhere on the forehead from the eyebrow to the hairline, with lower incisions providing the best predictability. With the "direct" approach, skin is removed immediately adjacent to the eyebrow, as in **Fig. 21**. This technique will reposition the eyebrow close to a 1:1 ratio for skin excision to eyebrow lift and therefore is arguably the most accurate eyebrow lift available. The primary disadvantage is a potentially visible scar, something that can be mitigated with patient selection and careful suture technique.[26–28]

A mid-brow approach can be used with an incision placed in a transverse forehead line, and the caudal side undermined and resected (**Fig. 22**). When a subcutaneous lift is attempted from the anterior hairline, the entire height of the forehead skin must be undermined. Although successful, the relapse problem is greater which necessitates more skin removal, possible as much as a 3:1 to 4:1 ratio for skin removal:eyebrow movement. To address this problem, the Gliding Browlift (GBL) has been described in which a blind undermining of the forehead skin is followed by shifting the skin and holding it in place with temporary, externally placed sutures. My own preference with this technique is to undermine the skin under direct vision through a 2 cm. incision. No skin is removed[29] (**Fig. 23**).

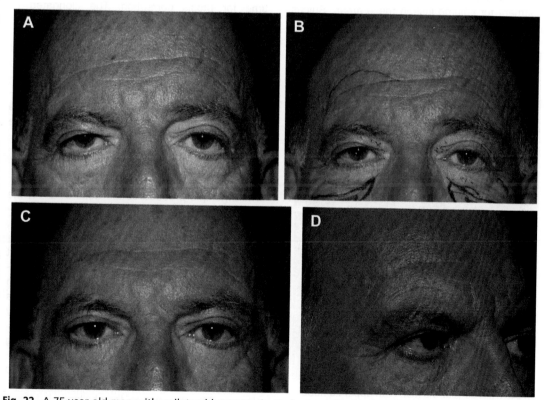

Fig. 22. A 75-year-old man with unilateral brow ptosis. He had a right-sided mid-brow subcutaneous brow lift, revision blepharoplasty, and fat grafting. (*A*) Preoperative view, (*B*) preoperative marking, (*C*) postoperative result at 6 months, and (*D*) forehead scar at 6 months.

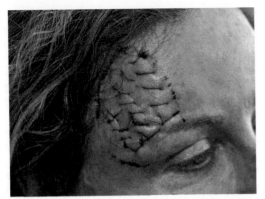

Fig. 23. A 45-year-old woman 1 day after a Gliding Browlift, done through an open incision. The dissection plane was on the frontalis muscle and after shifting the skin flap superiorly, externally placed sutures attach the skin to the frontalis at a higher level. The stitches were removed 3 days postoperatively.

FAT GRAFTING

A deficiency of soft tissue volume in the upper lid sulcus contributes to the appearance of hollow, elderly looking eyes. Similarly, loss of soft tissue around the supralateral orbital rim can lead to skeletal, aging appearance. Fat grafting is an excellent treatment for volume loss in these areas. Sulcus grafting has been described as "lowering the

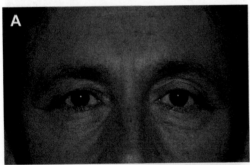

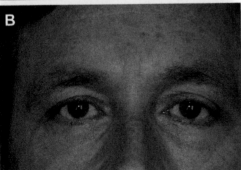

Fig. 24. (A) A 58-year-old man with upper lid hooding and a hollow left upper lid sulcus. (B) 1 year after an upper lid skin trim blepharoplasty and 2 cc of fat grafting to the left upper lid sulcus.

supraorbital rim" rather than filling the upper orbit with fat.[30] My technique closely follows that of Coleman.[31] The fat is harvested with a low-pressure syringe, using a harvesting cannula with small holes (1.5 mm) to keep the fat droplet size small. The fat is centrifuged for 1 minute to separate the layers and the fat is then injected with a blunt cannula with holes slightly larger than the harvesting holes (1.7 mm). Strategies to avoid injecting vessels include preinjecting the area with epinephrine containing local anesthetic and waiting long enough for the tissue to blanch—ensuring constriction of critical arteries. The injecting cannula should have a blunt tip with a side port and the injection should be done with low pressure. The cannula is kept moving to avoid a bolus injection in any one location. An example of upper sulcus fat grafting is shown in **Fig. 24**.

PTOSIS REPAIR

Upper lid ptosis cases of congenital, neurologic, or myogenic causes are typically treated by ophthalmologists using a tarsomullerectomy done through a conjunctival approach. Plastic surgeons typically encounter senile ptosis in older patients presenting for blepharoplasty. This is an ideal time for ptosis correction. The elongated or dehisced levator aponeurosis can be repaired with suture plication through an open blepharoplasty approach. It is helpful to have the patient awake enough to sit up before wound closure to confirm symmetry and the correct lid height. Adjustments are common. If a plastic surgeon is uncomfortable with ptosis repair, it should be referred to a colleague to be done ahead of time as a separate procedure.[32]

COMBINED SURGERY

When multiple procedures are done at once, the surgical order needs to be established. If fat grafting is planned, I prefer to do that at the beginning, before intraoperative edema from associated surgery sets in. If brow repositioning is planned, that should be done next, followed by upper lid blepharoplasty. Upper lid ptosis repair can be done in conjunction with blepharoplasty. Of course, as the number of variables increases, the complexity of the surgery increases.

The most common scenario for men requiring combined surgery is upper lid hooding in conjunction with a ptotic brow, or a brow that is likely to become ptotic after blepharoplasty (**Fig. 25**). In planning this combination, the challenge is to predict where the lifted eyebrows are likely to settle in the long term. Some brow lifts are more stable

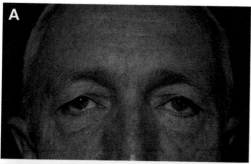

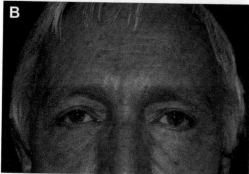

Fig. 25. (*A*) A 64-year-old man with lateral brow ptosis and upper lid soft tissue hooding. Neither blepharoplasty nor brow lift alone would provide adequate rejuvenation. (*B*) 8 months after an upper and lower lid blepharoplasty, a cutaneous brow lift using a mid-brow crease and fat grafting to his orbital rims, temples, and cheeks.

than others, whereas the soft tissue in some patients is more durable than in others. In this arena, experience is the best teacher. Over time, surgeons become familiar with the effect of certain procedures in certain types of patients—in their own hands. This knowledge allows for an informed decision about the amount of upper eyelid skin to be removed with simultaneous eyebrow repositioning.

When unsure about brow lift versus blepharoplasty, the brow lift can be done first, and after it has settled, over a period of 3 to 6 months, the blepharoplasty can be done with precision. Generally, with surgery in the male upper eyelid-brow junction, a conservative approach is safer because upper lid skin excision can easily be done later as a secondary procedure.

In treating the male upper lid-brow junction—less is always more.

CLINICS CARE POINTS

- Male eyebrows are lower and flatter than the female. In attractive men, the upper lid sulcus

is often a crowded space with minimal tarsal show.

- In response to upper lid hooding, men raise their eyebrows to clear their line of sight, resulting in transverse forehead lines.

- In seeking rejuvenation of the upper lid-brow junction, men want to look better. They do not want a stylized male appearance and they do not want to be feminized.

- At least one-third of men develop ptosis of their eyebrows and over 15% develop blepharoptosis.

- Men with hollowness of the upper lid sulcus can benefit from fat grafting.

- Brow lift surgery has a problem with the predictability of long-term results. This has resulted in many different techniques to elevate the eyebrows.

- Men are well suited to several different types of brow lift surgery, including endoscopic, direct cutaneous, and mid-brow cutaneous.

- In men with upper lid hooding and chronic frontalis contraction, an upper blepharoplasty, leads to frontalis relaxation and a lower eyebrow position.

- To prevent brow ptosis after blepharoplasty, a brow lift procedure is succesful if it stabilizes the brow in its preoperative location.

- In men, conservatism is the safest surgical philosophy at the upper lid-brow junction.

DISCLOSURE

The author has nothing to disclose.

REFERENCES

1. Westmore MG. Facial Cosmetics in conjunction with surgery. Course presented at Annual meeting of the American Society for aesthetic plastic surgery. Vancouver: British Columbia; 1975.
2. Gunter JP, Antrobus SD. Aesthetic analysis of the eyebrows. Plast Reconstr Surg 1997;99:1808–16.
3. Gülbitti HA, Bouman YK, Marten TJ, et al. The orbital oval balance principle: a morphometric clinical analysis. Plast Reconstr Surg 2018;142(4):451e–61e.
4. Marten TJ, Knize DM. Forehead aesethetics and preoperative assessment of the foreheadplasty patient. In: Knize DM, editor. The forehead and temporal Fossa anatomy and technique. Philadelphia: Lippincott Williams & Wilkins; 2001. p. 96–9.
5. Vaca EE, Bricker JT, Helenowsky I, et al. Identifying aesthetically appealing upper eyelid Topographic Proportions. Aesthet Surg J 2019;39(8):824–34.

6. Goldstein SM, Katowitz JA. The male eyebrow: a Topographic anatomic analysis. Ophthal Plast Reconstr Surg. 2005;21(4):285–91.

7. GQ.com.au. These are the Richest male models in the world. 2019.

8. Lambros V. Observations on periorbital and Midface aging. Plast Reconstr Surg 2007;120(5):1367–76.

9. Kahn DM, Shaw RB. Aging of the bony orbit. A Three-dimensional computed tomographic study. Aresthet Surg J 2008;28:258–64.

10. Sridharan GV, Tallis RC, Leatherbarrow B, et al. A community survey of ptosis of the eyelid and pupil size of elderly people. Age Ageing 1995;24:21–4.

11. Kim MH, Cho J, Zhao D, et al. Prevalence and associated factors of blepharoptosis in Korean adult population: the Korea National Health and Nutrition examination survey 2008–2011. Eye 2017;31:940–6.

12. Barsegian A, Botwinick A, Reddy HS. The phenylephrine test Revisited. Ophthal Plast Reconstr Surg 2018;34(2):151–4.

13. Chen AD, Lai YW, Lai HT, et al. The Impact of Hering's Law in blepharoptosis literature Review. Ann Plast Surg 2016;76:S96–100.

14. Carruthers JD, Carruthers JA. Treatment of glabellar frown lines with C. botulinum A exotoxin. J Dermatol Surg Oncol 1992;18(1):17–21.

15. Kane MAC. Nonsurgical periorbital and brow rejuvenation. Plast Reconstr Surg 2015;135(1):63–71.

16. Morley AMS, Taba M, Malhotra F, et al. Use of Hyaluronic Acid Gel for upper eyelid filling and Contouring. Ophthal Plast Reconstr Surg 2009;25(6):440–4.

17. Kontis CD, Rivkin A. The history of injectable facial fillers. Facial Plast Surg 2009;(2):67–72.

18. Fagien S. The role of the orbicularis oculi muscle and the eyelid crease in optimizing results in aesthetic upper blepharoplasty: a new look at the surgical treatment of mild upper eyelid fissure and fold asymmetries. Plast Reconstr Surg 2010;125(2):653–66.

19. Guyuron B, Son JH, Transpalpebral Corrugator Resection. 25-Year experience, Refinements and Additional indications. Aesthetic Plast Surg 2017; 41:339–45.

20. The aesthetic Society: Procedural Statistics. Available at: https://www.surgery.org/media/statistics. [Accessed 9 March 2021]. Accessed.

21. Core GB, Vasconez LO, Graham HD. Endoscopic browlift. Clin Plast Surg 1995;22(4):619–31.

22. Fisher O, Zamboni WA. Endoscopic brow-lift in the male patient. Arch Facial Plast Surg 2010;12:56–9.

23. Swift R, Nolan W, Basner A, et al. Endoscopic brow lift: objective results after 1 Year. Aesthet Surg J 1999;19(4):287–92.

24. Rohrich RJ, Cho MJ. Endoscopic temporal brow lift: surgical indications, technique, and 10-year Outcome analysis 2019;144(6):1305–10.

25. Warren RJ. The modified lateral brow lift. Aesthet Surg J 2009;29(2):158–66.

26. Castañares S. Forehead wrinkles, glabellar frown and ptosis of the eyebrows. Plast Reconstr Surg 1964;34:406–13.

27. Vinas JC, Caviglia C, Cortinas JL. Forehead rhytidoplasty and brow lifting. Plast Reconstr Surg 1976; 57(4):445–54.

28. Pelle-Ceravolo M, Angelini M. Transcutaneous brow shaping: a Straightforward and Precise method to lift and shape the eyebrows. Aesthet Surg J 2017; 37(8):863–75.

29. Viterbo F, Auersvald A, O'Daniel TG. Gliding brow lift (GBL): a new concept. Aesthetic Plast Surg 2019; 43:s1536–46.

30. Marten T, Personal communication, American Society for Aesthetic Plastic Surgery Annual Meeting. Teaching Course: Browlift. 2015.

31. Coleman SR. In: Structural fat grafting. St. Louis: Quality Medical Publishing Inc; 2019. p. 354-399.

32. Carraway JH, Tran P. Blepharoplasty with ptosis repair. Aesthet Surg J 2009;29:54–61.

Lower Lid Blepharoplasty in Men

Vinay Rao, MD, MPH[a], Patrick K. Sullivan, MD[b],*

KEYWORDS

• Lower lid • Blepharoplasty • Eyelid • Male • Facial rejuvenation • Aesthetics

KEY POINTS

- Lower lid blepharoplasty is a common aesthetic procedure in men.
- Changes at the lower lid secondary to aging involve the formation of deepened palpebromalar (lid-cheek junction) and nasojugal (tear-trough) grooves.
- Lower lid blepharoplasty using a transconjunctival technique may be preferred in men as it allows easy access to the periorbital fat compartments and nicely hides the surgical incision.
- Maneuvers to improve lower lid deformity include fat excision, orbitomalar ligament release with fat redraping, lower lid support/tightening procedures (canthopexies), and ancillary procedures such as skin resurfacing or autologous fat grafting to blend the lid-cheek junction.

OVERVIEW

A natural transition from the lower eyelid to the midface is paramount for a youthful facial appearance. Periorbital changes secondary to aging are often the first ones noticed by patients; therefore, optimizing lower eyelid contour is critical in facial rejuvenation. The eye exhibits an almond shape with fullness in the surrounding periorbital tissue, normal eyelid skin tone, smooth eyelid skin, and a slight upward tilt from the medial canthus to the lateral canthus.[1] The aging of the lower lid involves periorbital rhytid formation, pseudoherniation of periorbital fat, and lower eyelid laxity.[2] These changes represent the most common reasons why patients express dissatisfaction with their lower eyelid appearance.

The effects of aging on lower eyelid contour are similar across genders.[3] However, special consideration should be given during the surgical planning for lower lid blepharoplasties in men secondary to varying aesthetic norms and patient goals. Understanding the key distinguishing features in lower lid surgery for men is important, as it represents a common concern for male patients. In 2020, 14% of the blepharoplasties conducted in the US were done in men, amounting to the second most common cosmetic procedure performed in men following nose reshaping.[4]

Regardless of gender, lower lid blepharoplasty is recognized as one of the most challenging procedures to master in aesthetic surgery. In this article, the authors will review relevant lower eyelid anatomy, clinical assessment for the male patient, operative approach, postoperative complications, and the current evidence for lower lid blepharoplasties.

ANATOMY OF LOWER EYELID DEFORMITIES

A detailed understanding of both normal eyelid anatomy as well as the anatomic derivations to the changes seen with aging is critical in developing an effective and longstanding surgical result. The lower eyelid is composed of 3 lamellae—the anterior, middle, and posterior.[5] The anterior lamella is composed of skin and the orbicularis oculi muscle, the middle is composed of the orbital septum, and the posterior is made of the transligamentous sling and conjunctiva.[5] The transligamentous sling is the support structure for the lower eyelid and consists of the tarsal plate,

[a] Division of Plastic Surgery, The Warren Alpert Medical School of Brown University, 235 Plain Street, Suite 502, Providence, RI 02905, USA; [b] 235 Plain Street, Suite 502, Providence, RI 02905, USA
* Corresponding author.
E-mail address: cosmetic@drsullivan.com

Clin Plastic Surg 49 (2022) 213–220
https://doi.org/10.1016/j.cps.2021.12.001
0094-1298/22/© 2022 Elsevier Inc. All rights reserved.

capsulopalpebral fascia, and the canthal tendons.[5]

Among the anterior lamellae structures, the lower eyelid skin is the thinnest in the body and therefore is particularly prone to soft tissue changes that occur due to aging. The orbicularis oculi muscle lies just deep into the skin and is divided into the pretarsal, preseptal, and orbital components. The orbicularis muscle is a complex structure with 10 separate heads, consisting of both deep and superficial portions. It originates from the medial aspect of the orbit and inserts at the lateral aspect of the orbit.[6]

The orbital septum originates from the periosteal thickening of the orbital rim called the arcus marginalis.[7] In the lower eyelid, the septum fuses with the capsulopalpebral fascia superiorly and represents the anterior border for the periorbital fat compartments. There are 3 periorbital fat compartments, called the medial, central, and lateral compartment. The medial and central are demarcated by the inferior oblique muscle. The central and lateral are demarcated by an interpad septum and the arcuate expansion of Lockwood's lower lid suspensory ligament.[7]

The aging process affects all of these structures resulting in the typified periorbital senescent changes. In general, a youthful lower eyelid is vertically short with concavity over the orbital septum. The lower eyelid should smoothly transition to the convexity of the cheek, which is rounded from medial to lateral with maximal fullness and prominence over the zygoma.[2] Aging results in alterations to all the intricate structures of the lower eyelid. Lower eyelid skin thins, becomes dyspigmented, and periorbital rhytids develop. In addition, and perhaps the hallmark of aging lower eyelid, is the formation of a prominent palpebromalar groove (lid-cheek junction) and nasojugal groove (tear-trough deformity).[8]

The palpebromalar groove is a deep concavity that forms between the lower aspect of the lower eyelid and the cheek. A cadaveric study has suggested this demarcation as a natural cleft occurring between the bony attachments of the preseptal and orbital orbicularis oculi muscles.[9] This cleft is thought to become accentuated over time with periorbital fat pseudoherniation anteriorly through an attenuated orbital septum.[10] Alongside these changes, lower eyelid contour is further altered with midfacial fat atrophy and the descent of the malar fat mound.[11]

The orbital retaining ligament (ORL) is also important to consider when characterizing the palpebromalar groove. The ORL is distinct from the orbital septum and arises from the periosteum of the infraorbital rim and similarly is contiguous with the lateral orbital thickening and the superficial lateral canthal tendon.[12] Notably, the lower eyelid ORL functions as the caudal border of the lower eyelid fat compartments.[13] An intact ORL further contributes to a deepening palpebromalar groove as lower eyelid fat migrates and/or herniates through the orbital septum.

The nasojugal groove can be understood as the medial extension of the palpebromalar groove. Specifically, the nasojugal groove beings at the midpupillary line and medial to the extent of the medial canthus.[9] Similar to the palpebromalar groove, the tear trough deformity is thought to occur secondary to thinner skin in this area, cleft between the preseptal and orbital orbicularis oculi muscles, site of the origin of the medial extent of the preseptal orbicularis muscle at the maxilla below the infraorbital rim, and through accentuation with periorbital fat pseudoherniation and changes in the midface.[9] Overall, these anatomic features that occur with aging provide the basis for the tenets of surgical correction.

CLINICAL ASSESSMENT

Preoperative consultation should begin with discussing the patient's specific concerns and goals for surgery. Only after gaining a clear understanding of the patient's interests can the surgeon detail a customized surgical plan and properly guide patient expectations. Common lower eyelid complaints among male patients are the feeling of a tired facial appearance, sunken eyes, periorbital wrinkles, and lower lid skin looseness. Each of these issues should be targeted if surgical intervention is thought to be indicated.

A detailed medical history to ensure the patient is a good candidate for potential eyelid surgery should be obtained. Specific attention should be made to patients with a past medical history of hypertension, chronic dry eye symptoms, glaucoma, thyroid disease, and those on blood-thinning medications or herbal supplements. Past surgical history of prior lid procedures or recent ophthalmologic procedures should be clarified as repeat periorbital intervention may be unwarranted or should be delayed.

After a good history is obtained, a comprehensive physical examination focusing on the associated facial changes secondary to aging should be conducted. Visual acuity, periorbital sensation, voluntary and involuntary blink response, and normal extraocular muscle function should be confirmed. When examining the eye, the provider should also evaluate the position of the eye by noting the inferior position of the limbus to the lower eyelid margin and the degree of scleral show. From medial to lateral, the provider should assess for the presence of a prominent nasojugal groove, the extent of the palpebromalar groove, the descent and/or atrophy of the malar mound, and note any pseudoherniation or festooning of the periorbital fat compartments.

Orbital vector determination is another critical component of the preoperative evaluation.[1] Specifically, the globe position is evaluated in relation to the infraorbital rim. This relationship can best be seen in the lateral view of the patient. A neutral vector is defined as the cornea in line with the orbital rim and a positive vector is when the cornea is posterior to the rim. A negative vector, or when the cornea is anterior to the rim, increases the risk for postoperative ectropion, limiting the amount of periorbital fat excision that can be performed.[14]

In our patients, we find classifying patients based on the categories of lower lid deformities they may present with is extremely helpful in both surgical planning and patient education. We have identified 3 classes of lower lid abnormalities (**Fig. 1**). Type I is an isolated tear-trough deformity, Type II combines a tear-trough and a prominent lid-cheek deformity, and Type III is a combination deformity with excess periorbital fat. This conceptual model is helpful when evaluating patients; however, it is critical to offer a tailored approach based on the patient's specific needs. In general, for Type I and Type II patients, we do not remove skin and fat (except the lateral compartment), and, for Type III patients, we tend to remove fat from all 3 compartments.[15]

Integrity of the lateral canthal tendon should also be assessed independently. Lower lid laxity is critical to identity, as it represents a major contributor to the aged appearance of the lower eyelid.[16] This can be performed reliably using the distraction test. To perform this maneuver, the provider gently distracts the lower eyelid anteriorly until a distinct end point is felt. A distraction of greater than 10 mm is considered abnormal and often indicates lateral canthal tendon insufficiency. Additionally, the provider can simply pull down on the lower lid to assess canthal integrity. A lower lid displacement of more than 3 mm is considered abnormal. When a lax lower eyelid is diagnosed, a lid-shortening procedure should be planned.

SURGICAL TECHNIQUE

Surgical technique for lower lid blepharoplasty in men is not unlike in women. There have been numerous proposed techniques, each with its touted benefits. However, regardless of technique, the goal of lower lid blepharoplasty should be the same. That is, to restore a youthful lower eyelid appearance, achieved by smoothing the lid-cheek junction, filling the tear trough-deformity, and reducing the appearance of bulging fat in the lower eyelid.

The first major controversy in lower lid blepharoplasty technique is the placement of the incision. Some providers prefer to use a transcutaneous (subciliary) approach, which begins with a skin incision 1 mm below the lash line and 4 to 5 mm from the lateral canthal angle within an existing crow's foot. A skin-muscle flap is developed in the preseptal plane beneath the orbicularis oculi and carried down to the orbital rim. The critical step for this technique is the release of the ORL to allow for transposition of periorbital fat and smoothing of the palpebromalar groove. Additionally, the medial portion of the orbicular oculi muscle is detached from its origins in the presence of a tear-trough deformity to allow for the redistribution of fat into this defect.

We prefer a transconjunctival approach for accessing the periorbital fat compartments, emphasizing low complication rates and no visible scarring. We find this technique especially useful in men as complete fat redraping can be performed in patients with more severe deformities, and, as males often do not wear make-up, a hidden scar is even more critical for these patients. Preoperatively, in an upright position, the patient is carefully marked while in a neutral gaze. Each fat compartment is outlined as well as the palpebromalar and nasojugal grooves. The malar mound, if present, is also noted, as we need to ensure not to inadvertently enlarge this area during soft tissue manipulation and fat grafting procedures.

This technique is performed by designing a transconjunctival incision at 6 to 8 mm posterior to the lash line in the retroseptal position. The conjunctiva is divided using a fine point needle electrocautery. Once the conjunctiva is incised, dissection is carried down to the fat compartments that need treatment. If indicated the dissection is continued to the infraorbital rim in a blunt fashion through the capsulopalpebral fascia. The orbital septum and orbicularis oculi muscle are left undisturbed in this approach, which minimizes disruption to the connective tissue and preserves the vascularity of the flap.

Next, the ORL and the arcus marginalis can be released as needed with the dissection all being retroseptal. This maneuver allows for subsequent redraping of the periorbital fat and smoothing of a deepened orbitomalar sulcus and lid-cheek junction.[17,18] Dissection is carried further down in the subperiosteal plane using a Cottle elevator

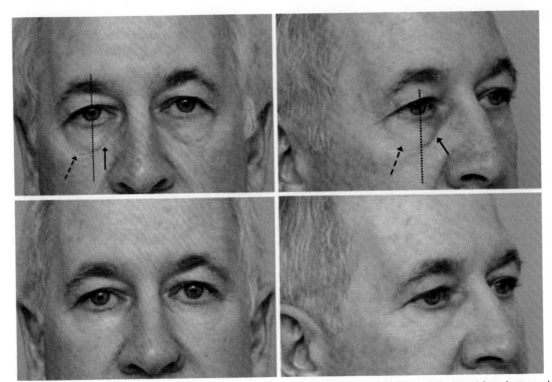

Fig. 1. Lower eyelid deformities associated with aging in a male. (Above) A 65-year-old man with a deepened palpebromalar groove with both s deep tear-trough deformity (*heavy arrow*) and a prominent lid-cheek junction (*dotted arrow*). (Below) His postoperative photos show improvement of these features. (*Courtesy of* Patrick K. Sullivan, MD, Providence, RI.)

with special care to release the dense attachments of the medial and lateral components of the pre-septal orbicularis oculi muscle to help correct for the nasojugal and palpebromalar deformities (**Fig. 2**).

The senior author (P.K.S.) prefers a transcon-junctival retroseptal approach because it leaves the orbital septum and orbicularis oculi intact. The fat compartments are easily accessed using this technique and periorbital fat excision can occur precisely, customized to the patient's need. Gentle pressure is placed on the upper eyelid over the globe, examining for bulging in any area to indicate under resection. Our preferred technique in men varies from more extensive release of the retaining orbitomalar ligaments (this is especially in the patient with a very negative vector) as described above (**Fig. 3**) to a less exten-sive targeted periorbital fat excision. This less extensive technique is used in patients who exhibit primarily fat excess and herniation. For most pa-tients, resolution of the palpebromalar and/or nasojugal deformities requires additional ancillary procedures of autologous fat grafting to fill areas of deficit to further help blend contour irregularities.

Patients with lid laxity need resuspension of the lower lid at the lateral canthus. If there is severe lid laxity (>6 mm of lower lid distraction), patients may require a lateral canthoplasty as previously described. In all other patients, a lateral cantho-pexy is often adequate to suspend, support, and tighten the lateral orbital soft tissue. We use a can-thopexy routinely and feel it has helped prevent lower lid malposition and scleral show.

We perform this procedure using a small upper eyelid incision in the natural crease with placement of a polydioxanone (5-0 PDS) suture between the inferior limb of the lateral canthal tendon and the periosteum of the lateral orbital rim. When placing this suture, the provider should confirm the lateral canthal tendon is grasped with gentle pull of the suture to confirm control of the lower eyelid. Place-ment of the stitch should achieve a gentle upward slant and contour of the lateral lower eyelid to globe. We do not overcorrect but rather place the lateral canthus in the optimal position. Finally, a lateral tarsorrhaphy suture is routinely used to help prevent the appearance of chemosis. That suture is usually removed on day 4.

After fat excision and/or redraping, and the lateral canthopexy excess skin can be addressed

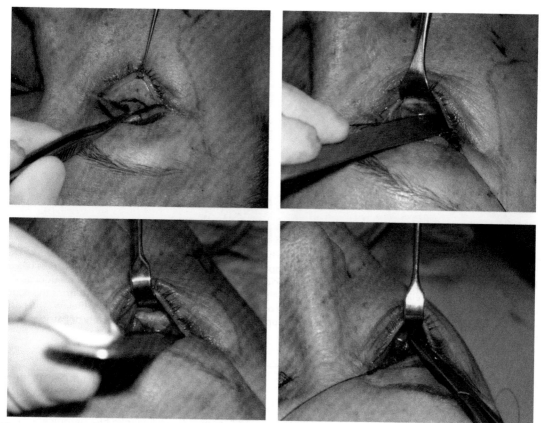

Fig. 2. Lower eyelid blepharoplasty using a transconjunctival retroseptal approach. (*Top Left*) Transconjunctival retroseptal incision designed 6-mm posterior to the lash line. (*Top Right*) Dissection through the capsulopalpebral fascia to expose the infraorbital rim and orbital retaining ligament. (*Bottom Left*) Release of the orbital retaining ligament to expose the infraorbital rim in the subperiosteal plane. (*Bottom Right*) Exposure of periorbital fat with redraping along the lid-cheek junction and suture fixation. (*Courtesy of* Patrick K. Sullivan, MD, Providence, RI.)

using a careful pinch technique. In our experience, we find that excess skin resection is rarely needed for lower eyelid blepharoplasty once the appropriate amount of fat is removed and redistributed. Chemical peels and laser resurfacing are also treatments we use to address skin aging.

COMPLICATIONS

The most feared complication following blepharoplasty Is vision loss by retrobulbar hematoma, which has been reported in less than 0.05% of cases and most frequently occurs intraoperatively or within the first 24 hours postoperatively.[19] We have never had blindness or loss of vision in any of our hundreds of lower lid surgeries. Other early complications include corneal abrasion, infection, hematoma, and chemosis. In lower lid blepharoplasty, lid malposition can also be a problem. This complication can effectively be avoided with careful preoperative clinical assessment to characterize the presence and severity of lower lid laxity. Choosing the correct lower lid resuspension technique, either canthoplasty or canthopexy, is an important step to properly position the lower lid in the optimal position.

CURRENT EVIDENCE

The senior author previously performed a comprehensive review regarding the current evidence regarding lower blepharoplasty techniques.[20] One of the major considerations in lower lid blepharoplasty is the decision between performing a transconjunctival or transcutaneous approach. For transconjunctival approaches, many authors have argued for aggressive ligamentous release to properly redistribute periorbital fat and blend the lower lid with the midface.[20] In these cases, the fat can either be preserved and transposed or conservatively resected. Excess skin resected using the skin pinch technique has been

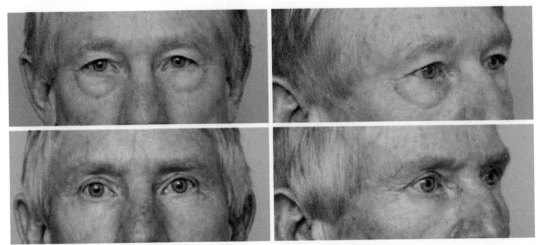

Fig. 3. Case example of the senior author's preferred technique for lower lid blepharoplasty in men. (Above) This is a 60-year-old-man who presented with redundant upper eyelid skin and was concerned with puffiness below the eyes. A skin-only resection of the upper lids was performed. The patient exhibited significant pseudohernia- tion of fat at the lower eyelid resulting in a deepened palpebromalar and nasojugal groove. To address this issue, a transconjunctival retroseptal approach was used with conservative fat excision and redraping. (Below) The post- operative photos show significant improvements in the upper and lower lid aesthetics. (*Courtesy of* Patrick K. Sul- livan, MD, Providence, RI.)

demonstrated as effective, as providers can take advantage of the absence of undermining and can even use laser resurfacing procedures as an adjunct. Authors have reported a good to excellent success rate performing these combined techniques.[21]

Others have reported on their experience with the transconjunctival approach and saw satisfac- tory results when assessing for various objective measures such as pupil to eyelid margin, pupil to tear trough distance, tear trough width, and changes at the intercanthal angles without any major complications.[22] Hidalgo and colleagues published a series of 248 patients undergoing their particular lower lid approach using transconjuncti- val access, reporting excellent outcomes and a 2.4% revision rate.[23]

Transcutaneous approaches have been associ- ated with malposition at a rate anywhere between 15% and 20%, orbicularis denervation atrophy, and a 1% rate of possible frank ectropion in some series.[23,24] Authors have argued that trans- cutaneous access allows for more aggressive liga- ment release allowing for more definitive treatment of severe deformities. Barton and colleagues described their technique of a transcutaneous ac- cess and a broad orbital retaining ligament release in 71 patients with severe deformities, illustrating excellent results and 1 patient suffering from lower lid malposition.[25] For some authors, the additional benefit of a transcutaneous approach is the ability to perform a suborbicularis oculi fat (SOOF) lift.

Using a SOOF-lift, authors contend that there is an increased ability to blend the lid-cheek junction by redraping this fat over the orbital rim.[26]

Still, conventional lower lid blepharoplasty, con- sisting of skin-muscle flap technique and without fat resection or transposition or midfacial proced- ures, remains a popular choice for some providers. Maffi and colleagues reported outcomes on 2007 lower lid procedures using this approach, yielding excellent results and only a 0.04% lower lid malpo- sition rate.[27]

SUMMARY

Lower lid blepharoplasty is a critical technique to master as it remains an important aesthetic concern for men. Lower lid techniques vary but center around addressing the consequences of aging, including the formation of a deep palpebro- malar groove and tear-trough deformity. There is limited literature available publishing on clinical outcomes relating to lower lid blepharoplasty in men, in particular. In our experience, the anatomy of the aging eyelid is somewhat similar across gen- ders. As a result, providers can use standard tech- niques involving either skin-muscle flap, orbital retaining ligament release, fat transposition, fat excision, and/or midfacial filling procedures. Pro- viders may prefer using transconjunctival access in men to best hide the incision and still provide periorbital rejuvenation. We have found fat injec- tions to be a particularly helpful adjunct to lower lid blepharoplasty in rejuvenation of the male lower eyelid, lid-cheek junction, and cheek abnormalities.

CLINICS CARE POINTS

- Assess orbital vector during your preclinical assessment to ensure the appropriate surgical plan is chosen
- Grade the severity of lower lid laxity as most patients will require lid tightening or shortening procedures
- Transconjunctival approach should be designed in the retroseptal plane to preserve the orbital septum and provide direct access to the periorbital fat compartments
- Be careful not to over resect when removing periorbital fat as this may create an unnatural, hollowed out appearance to the eye
- Targeted periorbital fat excision along with autologous fat grafting to the lid-cheek junction may be all that's needed to provide an optimal result for the male patients

DISCLOSURE

The authors have no relevant financial disclosures.

REFERENCES

1. Jelks GW, Jelks EB. Preoperative evaluation of the blepharoplasty patient: Bypassing the pitfalls. Clin Plast Surg 1993;20:213–23.
2. Mendelson BC. Fat preservation technique of lower-lid blepharoplasty. Aesthet Surg J 2001;21:450–9.
3. Barrera JE, Most SP. Management of the lower lid in male blepharoplasty. Facial Plast Surg Clin North Am 2008;16:313–6.
4. American Society for Aesthetic Plastic Surgery. Cosmetic surgery National Data bank: Statistics 2012. Available at: https://www.plasticsurgery.org/documents/News/Statistics/2020/cosmetic-procedures-men-2020.pdf. Accessed September 5, 2021.
5. Muzaffar AR, Mendelson BC, Adams WP Jr. Surgical anatomy of the ligamentous attachments of the lower lid and lateral canthus. Plast Reconstr Surg 2002;110:873–84.
6. Loeb R. Aesthetic surgery of the eyelids. New York: Springer-Verlag; 1989.
7. Nahai F. The Art Aesthetic Surgery: Principles and Techniques. St. Louis, Missouri; 2nd edition; 2011.
8. Hamra ST. The role of the septal reset in creating a youthful eyelid-cheek complex in facial rejuvenation. Plast Reconstr Surg 2004;113:2124–41.
9. Haddock NT, Saadeh PB, Boutros S, et al. The tear trough and lid/cheek junction: anatomy and implications for surgical correction. Plast Reconstr Surg 2009;123:1332–40.
10. Tomlinson FB, Hovey LM. Transconjunctival lower lid blepharoplasty for removal of fat. Plast Reconstr Surg 1975;56:314–8.
11. Mendelson BC, Muzaffar AR, Adams WP Jr. Surgical anatomy of the midcheek and malar mounds. Plast Reconstr Surg 2002;110:885–96.
12. Ghavami A, Pessa JE, Janis J, et al. The orbicularis retaining ligament of the medial orbit: Closing the circle. Plast Reconstr Surg 2008;121:994–1001.
13. Rohrich RJ, Pessa JE. The fat compartments of the face: anatomy and clinical implications for cosmetic surgery. Plast Reconstr Surg 2007;119:2219–27 [discussion 2228–31].
14. Pessa JE, Desvigne LD, Zadoo VP. Changes in ocular globetoorbital rim position with age: implications for aesthetic blepharoplasty of the lower eyelids. Aesthet Plast Surg 1999;23:337–42.
15. Sullivan PK, Drolet BC. Extended lower lid blepharoplasty for eyelid and midfacial rejuvenation. Plast Reconstr Surg 2013;132(5):1093–101.
16. Rankin B, Arden R, Crumley R. Lower eyelid blepharoplasty. 2nd edition. New York: Thieme; 2002.
17. Pacella SJ, Nahai FR, Nahai F. Transconjunctival blepharoplasty for upper and lower eyelids. Plast Reconstr Surg 2010;125:384–92.
18. Hamra ST. Arcus marginalis release and orbital fat preservation in midface rejuvenation. Plast Reconstr Surg 1995;96:354–62.
19. Hass AN, Penne RB, Stefanyszyn MA, et al. Incidence of postblepharoplasty orbital hemorrhage and associated visual loss. Ophthal Plast Reconstr Surg 2004;20:426–32.
20. Drolet BC, Sullivan PK. Evidence-based medicine: blepharoplasty. Plast Reconstr Surg 2013;133(132):1195–205.
21. Kim EM, Bucky LP. Power of the pinch: pinch lower lid blepharoplasty. Ann Plast Surg 2008;60(5):532–7.
22. Rohrich RJ, Ghavami A, Mojallal A. The five-step lower blepharoplasty: blending the eye-lid cheek junction. Plast Reconstr Surg 2011;128(3):775–83.
23. Hidalgo DA. An integrated approach to lower blepharoplasty. Plast Reconstr Surg 2011;127:386–95.
24. Rosenberg DB, Lattman J, Shah AR. Prevention of lower eyelid malposition after blepharoplasty: anatomic and technical considerations of the inside-out blepharoplasty. Arch Facial Plast Surg 2007;9:434–8.

25. Barton FE Jr, Ha R, Awada M. Fat extrusion and septal reset in patients with the tear trough triad: a critical appraisal. Plast Reconstr Surg 2004;113: 2115–21.

26. Rohrich RJ, Arbique GM, Wong C, et al. The anatomy of suborbicularis fat: implications for periorbital rejuvenation. Plast Reconstr Surg 2009;124(3): 946–51.

27. Maffi TR, Chang S, Friedland JA. Traditional lower blepharoplasty: is additional support necessary? A 30 year review. Plast Reconstr Surg 2011;128: 265–73.

Male Facelift

Timothy Marten, MD*, Dino Elyassnia, MD

KEYWORDS

- Facelift • Male facelift • SMAS • High SMAS • Facelift incisions

KEY POINTS

- Male facial aesthetics differ from those in female patients and attractive masculinity is not as closely correlated with youth and beauty in male patients, and men generally seek a somewhat different outcome from facial rejuvenation surgery than do women.
- A well-contoured neck is an artistic imperative to an attractive and appealing masculine appearance, and a bold, well-defined neck and jawline conveys a sense of youth, health, fitness, strength, and vitality.
- Neck improvement is of high priority to almost every male patient, and the results of male facelift procedures are often largely judged by the outcome achieved in the neck. If the neck is not sufficiently improved, most male patients believe their surgeon has failed them.
- It is not possible to design or use a universal male facelift technique because each male patient presents with a unique set of problems that require precise anatomic diagnosis and an appropriately planned and individualized surgical repair.
- Committed study, careful planning, and avoiding the use of a cookie-cutter formula technique maximizes improvement, and minimizes problems and complications.

AGING OF THE MALE FACE AND MALE FACIAL AESTHETICS

Treatment strategies in men are different than those in women and it is not appropriate to arbitrarily apply concepts and techniques that evolved largely for treating women to men. Rejuvenation of the male face is arguably more nuanced than that of a female, whom society has come to accept as having a more contrived and made-up appearance, and certain aspects of male facial aging are often regarded as signs of experience, wisdom, and power that many men wish not to lose. In these and other ways men often have different goals than women do when seeking rejuvenation of their faces, with the man arguably more concerned about a natural appearance free of signs that a surgical procedure has been performed.[1] If one sees a woman whose face shows signs suggesting that a facelift might have been performed, one smiles and infers "she has had something done." If one sees a man with telltale signs that surgery has been performed, one is often more judgmental and disapproving. Women, who typically wear longer hairstyles and makeup, also have more ways to hide signs that surgery has been performed than a man. In this sense, there is perhaps arguably less room for error, technically and artistically, when a male facelift is performed.

In the current cultural climate female attractiveness is seen as correlated with smooth skin, a wrinkleless forehead, an arched eyebrow, a stylized eye appearance, a high cheek profile, a tight jawline, and overall inverted oval facial shape. Male attractiveness, however, is correlated with a more bottom heavy rectangular facial shape, a heavier and bolder jawline, a strong athletic neckline, a lower and more horizontal eyebrow, a flatter cheek profile, and less meticulously maintained skin. When these differences are contemplated it is seen that a different end point is often sought by men seeking facelift surgery, and the goals of the procedure and accompanying technique must be modified accordingly.

Men primarily seek and desire a bold, athletic neck and jawline, and more subtle and less

Marten Clinic of Plastic Surgery, 450 Sutter Street, Suite 2222, San Francisco, CA 94108, USA
* Corresponding author.
E-mail address: tmarten@martenclinic.com

Clin Plastic Surg 49 (2022) 221–256
https://doi.org/10.1016/j.cps.2021.12.005
0094-1298/22/© 2022 Elsevier Inc. All rights reserved.

dramatic changes on other areas of the face. All things considered, a surgeon who can deliver a good result in the neck and jawline, provide well-concealed scars, and exercise restraint when operating on the forehead, eyes and mouth, is likely to be successful when treating male patients. In contrast, surgeons who overtreat the orbital area, do not provide well-concealed scars, and do not deliver a good result in the neck are likely to have more unhappy male patients.

Recognizing the Components of the Aging Deformity of the Face

Recognizing the components of the aging deformity of the face, appreciating the underlying anatomic abnormalities, and understanding how men seek a somewhat different aesthetic end point than women is essential to properly advising patients and fundamental to the planning of any surgical procedure. Careful analysis reveals that most patient problems fall into three broad categories: (1) aging and breakdown of the skin surface; (2) facial sagging, skin redundancy, and loss of youthful facial contour; and (3) facial atrophy and/or age-related lipodystrophy. Proper treatment depends on the types of problems present; the patient's priorities; and the time, trouble, and expense he is willing to endure to obtain the desired improvement.[2–4]

Male patients are often less concerned with *surface aging* of their face and as such infrequently request or require dermatologic surface treatments of the skin. Men more often are primarily concerned with facial sagging, skin excess, and *loss of facial contour* and achieve little improvement if surface treatments of the skin only are used. They as a result more typically request and require formal surgical lifts in which sagging tissue is repositioned and redundant tissue is excised if these problems are to be properly corrected and an attractive and natural-appearing improvement is to be obtained.

Many of the changes associated with loss of facial contour in men represent primarily deep layer problems that are inadequately corrected if traditional skin-only facelift and neck lift techniques are used.[5] Regrettably, many surgeons unfamiliar with deep layer techniques,[6–8] and other physicians insufficiently trained to perform them, often use a variety of conceptually flawed procedures including skin-only "mini-lifts," "suture lifts," and noninvasive "skin shrinking" procedures and resort to other misguided and misapplied ancillary procedures to overcome the shortcomings of these methods in men. Although ancillary procedures are at times indicated in male patients, they are unnecessary in most cases if a superficial musculoaponeurotic system (SMAS) facelift and deep layer rejuvenation is performed (**Fig. 1**).[9–11]

Male patients frequently present at older ages than women and have significant *facial atrophy* and age-related loss of facial volume, and as a result generally achieve suboptimal improvement from surface treatments of facial skin and surgical lifts. Smoothing skin does not hide a drawn appearance caused by loss of facial volume, and it is difficult to create natural and masculine contours by lifting and repositioning tissues that have abnormally thinned and deflated with age. Restoring lost facial volume with autologous fat grafting[2–4] is a powerful technique that is increasingly being recognized as important in treating the aging male face. Properly performed, the addition of fat to areas of the male face that have atrophied because of age or disease can produce a significant and sustained improvement in appearance unobtainable by other means (see **Fig. 1**; **Figs. 37–39**; **Figs. 40-43**; **Figs. 44–48**). When an SMAS facelift technique is used in conjunction with fat grafting loss of facial contour and facial atrophy are corrected and optimal improvement in the male patient's appearance is obtained.

TREATMENT STRATEGIES IN THE MALE PATIENT

There are several situations one encounters in treating men in which a somewhat different strategy should be used than one would use in women.

The Bald Man and the Man with Short Hair

The bald man or the man with short hair, although often regarded by some surgeons as a significant challenge, can in reality be treated largely the way a man or woman with abundant hair is treated. Even sparse, short hair provides good cover for the temple (see **Figs 8**, **30**, **36**) and occipital incisions (see **Figs 2**, **17**, **20**) if properly planned and carried out because the short hair worn by most men falls over them and conceals them. This is the case even in the man who wears a military-style haircut. In these patients the basic facelift incision plan need not be specifically modified (**Figs. 2** and **8**. see also **Figs. 37–39**, **40–43**, and **44–48**).

Small incision and endoscopic foreheadplasty[12] is also usually possible in these patients if indicated because incisions are sited on the temple scalp and at the superior-most spot that hair is present (**Fig. 26**; **Figs. 44–48**). Alternatively, a forehead lift is performed by excising forehead skin along a transverse forehead crease (**Fig. 28**), or by using a supraciliary "direct eyebrow lift" incision

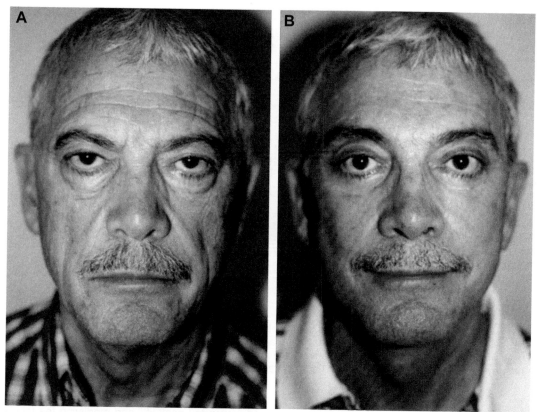

Fig. 1. Male Facelift Patient. (*A*) Before surgery view of patient, age 59. He is seen to have combined surface aging of his skin, tissue sagging and redundancy, and facial atrophy. Note heavily wrinkled forehead, hollow cheeks, deep cheek folds, and sagging facial tissues. (*B*) Same patient, 1 year and 6 months after facelift, neck lift, forehead lift, upper blepharoplasty with levator reinsertion, lower blepharoplasty, and facial fat grafting. Note improvement in forehead wrinkling, brow position, eye appearance, lower eyelid fullness, posture of perioral tissues, and overall facial sagging. Increased facial fullness following fat grafting is also evident. The patient has a more youthful, healthy, and masculine appearance without a tight, pulled, or face lifted look. All surgical procedures performed by Timothy Marten, MD, FACS. (*Courtesy of* Timothy Marten, MD, FACS, San Francisco, CA)

plan (**Fig. 29**).[13–15] Both these strategies result in inconspicuous scars if carried out correctly and represent a worthwhile trade-off in most men in the facelift age group.

Man with Shaved Head

Although once an oddity, the shaved head has become a near cultural norm and an increasingly common fashion statement, and this has resulted in plastic surgeons encountering a growing number of these men seeking facelifts and related procedures. Although these patients may initially present a quandary and are often turned away by many surgeons, they are good candidates for facelift surgery if a thoughtful surgical plan is used.

In treating the man with the shaved head one can exploit the fact that a key and quintessential feature of an attractive, athletic-appearing man is a good neckline. Unlike women, for whom optimal appearances are more closely tied to youth, an inverted oval facial shape, high cheek contour, and a tight jawline, the male face is more tolerant of a rectangular shape, a lower cheek profile, and a lax jawline. As such, a short scar neck lift[16] (neck lift using a submental incision only) performed in conjunction with ancillary procedures, such as fat grafting,[2–4] superciliary direct eyebrow lift, nasolabial fold excision, and conservative eyelid surgery, can result in satisfactory improvement without the need for a full facelift and periauricular scars (**Fig. 3**).

In a short scar neck lift a submental incision only is used and improved neck contour is obtained by treatment of deep layer neck structures and not the excision of neck skin. These deep layer treatments include subplatysmal lipectomy, submandibular gland reduction, partial digastric myectomy, and platysmaplasty. Skin is then allowed to redrape over the deeper and

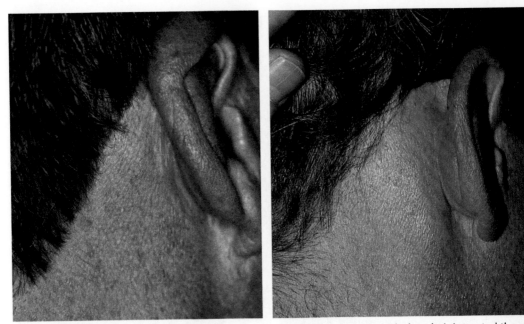

Fig. 2. Occipital hairline scar in men with short hair. The bald man or the man with short hair is treated the way a man or woman with abundant hair is treated. Even sparse, short hair provides good cover for the temple and occipital incisions if properly planned as is seen in the postoperative patients. Surgical procedures performed by Timothy Marten, MD, FACS. (*Courtesy of* Timothy Marten, MD, FACS, San Francisco, CA)

geometrically longer concave surface created and this, in effect, takes up loose neck skin. Short scar neck lift is productive in men well into their 60s in most cases (**Fig. 4**).

If a man with a shaved head believes excess skin is present that needs to be removed an extended neck lift[5,7] incision plan is used (typical periauricular facelift incision with a short or no temporal portion) (**Fig. 5**) modified by shortening or eliminating the occipital portion of the incision. Typically men needing and requesting this are older (in their 60s or 70s) and the scar is less of an issue and better concealed on their more aged skin than in the typical short scar candidate (30s to 60s).

The Facelift Phobic Man

Many men are put off by the word "facelift" and even when their typical fears of "looking different," "having a pulled or tight appearance," or "having obvious scars" are countered with explanations as to how those occurrences can be avoided, it is difficult to convince them to undergo the procedure. Often it seems that they want the improvement afforded by the facelift but just cannot get past the name of the procedure. In such cases an accord can usually be struck and the patient is accommodated by simply calling the procedure

an "extended neck lift" and modifying the facelift incision plan slightly accordingly.

In the extended neck lift a typical periauricular facelift incision is used but a short or no temporal portion of the incision is made (see **Fig. 5**). Such a plan places the incision and resulting scar in a well-concealed location but negates the possibility of a poorly concealed scar in the temporal area or sideburn retrodisplacement. This incision plan allows a limited low cheek SMAS flap to be elevated (or a low cheek SMAS plication or SMAS stacking procedure or the like to be performed) as part of the procedure that provides improvement in the lower face and along the jawline that would not otherwise be obtained if an isolated neck lift only was performed. In addition, it allows the excision of a significant amount of skin from the lower face, jawline, and neck that would not otherwise be removed. It should be noted that the extended neck lift encompasses certain compromises, however, including that no upper cheek or midface improvement is obtained. Although this is often an unacceptable compromise when operating on the female face, it is an acceptable trade-off in the male patient.

The extended neck lift is combined with fat grafting to offset some of its limitations and to obtain improvement on the upper face. Conservatively performed forehead and eyelid surgery

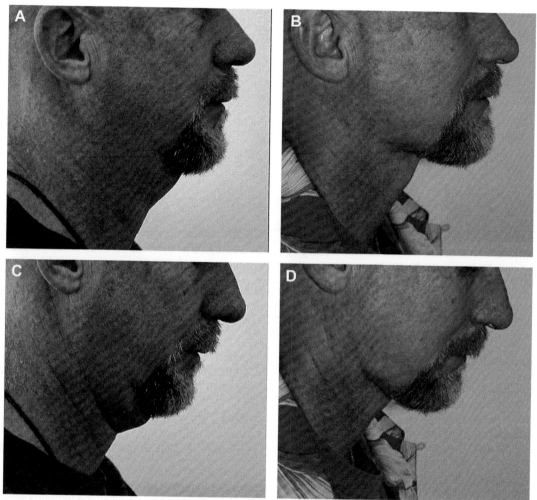

Fig. 3. Short scar neck lift in patient with a shaved head. (*A* and *C*) Patient before surgery. (*B* and *D*) Same patient after short scar neck lift (no skin excision). A submental incision only is used and improved neck contour is obtained by modification of deep layer neck structures and not the excision of neck skin. Skin is then allowed to redrape and redistribute itself over the deeper and geometrically longer concave surface created and this takes up loose neck skin. No scar is present around or behind the ear (see also **Fig. 4**). This strategy works well for the man with a shaved head who requests a facelift. All surgical procedures performed by Timothy Marten, MD. (*Courtesy of* Timothy Marten, MD, FACS, San Francisco, CA)

(discussed previously and later) can further enhance the outcome.[13]

Short Scar Facelifts in Man

A traditional short scar incision plan offers little benefit for most men and can in reality be problematic in many cases. The basic premise of shifting facial skin strongly in a vertical direction is conceptually flawed and typically results in the need for aggressive temple or forehead lifts and tedious gathering of redundancy along a temporal hairline incision that might not otherwise be required. Gathering of tissue, and the often corresponding puckering and bunching of skin along

incisions in the temple and postlobular areas that typically occurs when short scar incision plans are used, are concealed to some extent by women who typically wear longer hairstyles, but is a significant source of embarrassment to men (**Fig. 6**). Vertical skin shifts can also move deep cervical wrinkles from the neck up onto the lower face, a problem not encountered when a postauricular incision is used and a proper, more posteriorly directed vector for skin shift is used. In addition, because neck improvement is of paramount importance in men, it could be argued that shortening the scar in the postauricular area where it should be well concealed even in a man with short

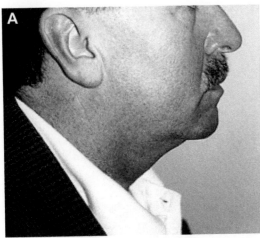
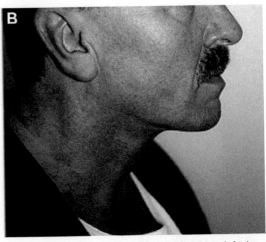

Fig. 4. Short scar neck lift. (*A*) Patient before surgery. (*B*) Same patient after short scar neck lift. His weight is un-changed. He has a more fit, healthy, decisive, and masculine appearance despite that no procedures have been performed elsewhere on his face. A submental incision only is used and improved neck contour is obtained by modification of deep layer neck structures and not the excision of neck skin. Skin is then allowed to redrape and redistribute itself over the deeper and geometrically longer concave surface created and this takes up loose neck skin. No scar is present around or behind the ear. All surgical procedures performed by Timothy Marten, MD, FACS. (*Courtesy of* Timothy Marten, MD, FACS, San Francisco, CA)

hair (see **Fig. 2**, **Figs. 40–43 Figs. 44–48**), and compromising overall result in the cervical region, is conceptually flawed and of dubious value.

Shortening the occipital portion of the facelift incision may be useful and a worthwhile compro-mise, however, in the man with the shaved head (see previous discussion).

PREOPERATIVE PLANNING IN THE MALE FACELIFT PATIENT

It is not possible to design or use a universal male facelift technique because each male patient pre-sents with a unique set of problems that require precise anatomic diagnosis and an appropriately

planned and individualized surgical repair. Committed study, careful planning, and avoiding the use of a formula technique maximize improve-ment, limit secondary irregularities, and minimize complications.

Planning Incisions in the Male Facelift Patient

Planning the temple incision
The temporal portion of the facelift incision has traditionally been placed within the temporal scalp in a well-intended, but all too frequently counter-productive attempt to hide the resulting scar. When cheek skin redundancy is small and abun-dant temple and sideburn hair is present, such a

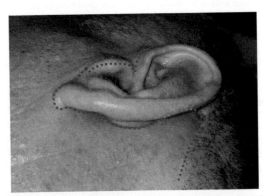

Fig. 5. Extended neck lift incision plan. The incision plan for an extended neck lift is similar to the typical peri-auricular facelift incision plan without the temporal portion of the incision. This incision plan allows lower facial skin to be excised and a low SMAS flap to be elevated and advanced or low SMAS plication to be performed that provides improvement in the lower face and along the jawline that would not otherwise be obtained if an iso-lated neck lift only was performed. (*Courtesy of* Timothy Marten, MD, FACS, San Francisco, CA)

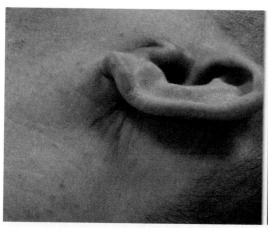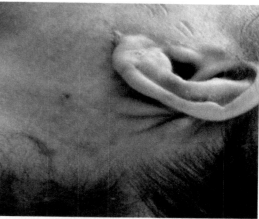

Fig. 6. Flawed short scar facelift incision plans. A short scar incision plan offers little benefit to most men and is problematic in many cases. Gathering of tissue, and the often resulting puckering and bunching of skin along incisions in the temple and postauricular areas that typically occurs when short scar incision plans are used, is concealed to some extent by women who typically wear longer hairstyles, but are a significant source of embarrassment to men. Procedures performed by unknown surgeons. (*Courtesy of* Timothy Marten, MD, FACS, San Francisco, CA)

plan is used without producing objectionable sideburn elevation and temporal hairline displacement (**Fig. 7**).

This, however, is often not the case for male patients who typically present for facelifts at a later age. Patients best suited for this incision plan are usually younger men who are troubled by mild to moderate cheek laxity only. In older men, however, skin shifts and the presence of sparse temple hair can result in unnatural, telltale, and effeminate-appearing displacement of the temporal hairline and sideburn if such a plan is used. Proper analysis, careful planning, and the use of an incision along the hairline, when indicated, can avert this problem without compromising the overall outcome of the procedure (**Figs. 8**, **9**, and **44–48).**[17]

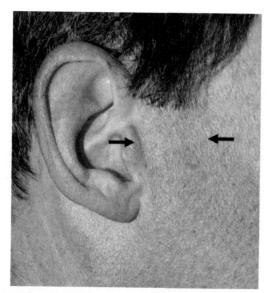

Fig. 7. Temple scalp temporal incision plan. When cheek skin redundancy is small and abundant temple and sideburn hair is present, an incision hidden in the temple scalp (*red dotted line*) is used without producing objectionable sideburn and temporal hairline displacement. Note sideburn and bearded skin in front of the ear (*area between black arrows*) have been moved posteriorly closer to the ear as a result of this patient's surgery, but not objectionably so. Note also the shift of some bearded skin onto the tragus. Procedure performed by Timothy Marten, MD, FACS. (*Courtesy of* Timothy Marten, MD, FACS, San Francisco, CA)

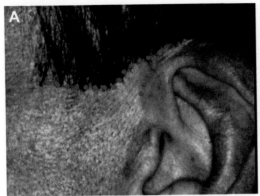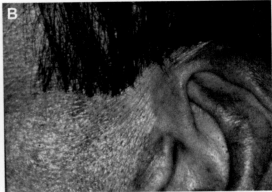

Fig. 8. Temporal hairline incision in the male patient. (*A*) Plan for temple hairline incision in the male patient. Note that unlike the incision plan in a female patient that is made as a soft curve, the incision in men should be planned in a more angular fashion echoing the shape of the male sideburn. (*B*) Close-up of postoperative healed incision. Hairline displacement has been avoided and the scar is well concealed. The sideburn has an angular masculine shape and has not been retrodisplaced or diminished in size. Procedure performed by Timothy Marten, MD, FACS. (*Courtesy of* Timothy Marten, MD, FACS, San Francisco, CA)

This incision accommodates large posterior-superior skin flap shifts and allows maximum improvement in the upper lateral face to be made. If it is made with care and closed under no tension, the resulting scar is usually inconspicuous and is far less obvious and troublesome for the patient than a displaced hairline. This is particularly true for men whose temple hair is generally kept cut short and usually falls forward and over the scar as opposed to women who typically wear their hair long and tuck it up over their ear

exposing the scar. The length of the temple-sideburn incision is varied depending of the amount of redundant skin in the upper lateral cheek, and the amount of midface improvement obtained (see **Fig. 9**).

Planning the preauricular incision

Open to inspection, the preauricular region exists as a frequent point of reference for those seeking to identify a facelift patient. Traditionally, incisions in this area in men are made well anterior to the

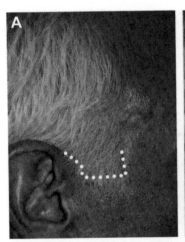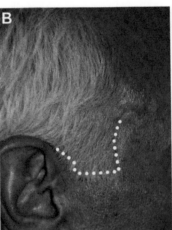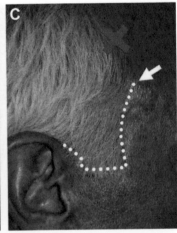

Fig. 9. Length of the temple hairline incision. The superior extent of temporal hairline incision varies depending on the amount of cheek skin shift predicted (and whether a forehead lift is to be concomitantly performed) if puckering and gathering is to be avoided in this area. (*A*) Superior extent of temple hairline incision when modest cheek skin displacement is predicted (*dotted line*). (*B*) Superior extent of temple hairline incision when moderate cheek skin displacement is predicted (*dotted line*). The incision must be made higher to accommodate the cheek skin shift, but still is situated in a well-concealed location. (*C*) Superior extent of temple hairline incision when large cheek skin displacement is predicted (*dotted line*). This incision should be made no higher than the junction of the temporal hairline with the frontotemporal hairline (*point shown by arrow*). If it is carried more superiorly along the frontotemporal hairline (*area designated by X*) the resulting scar is usually visible because hair tends to grow posteriorly in that area. Procedure performed by Timothy Marten, MD, FACS. (*Courtesy of* Timothy Marten, MD, FACS, San Francisco, CA)

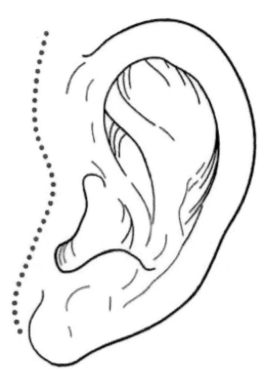

Fig. 10. Traditional location of the preauricular incision. This incision plan places the scar in most men in an area open to inspection by others and "brands" the patient as having had facelift surgery. Gradients of color and texture between smooth, pale auricular skin and coarse cheek skin draw additional attention to the scar (see **Fig. 11** AB). (*Courtesy of* Timothy Marten, MD, FACS, San Francisco, CA.)

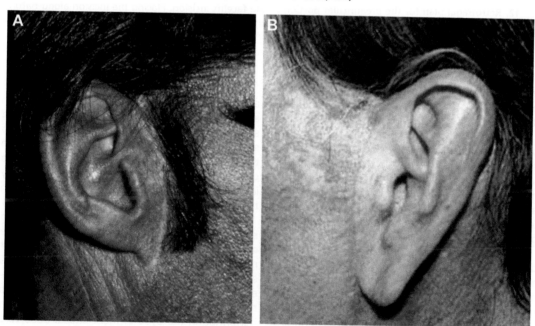

Fig. 11. Typical irregularities seen when a pretragal incision is used in male patients. (*A*) An unknown surgeon has mistakenly tried to hide the preauricular incision in a pretragal location along the posterior border of bearded skin. The scar is easily seen in the exposed location and a gradient of color and texture on each side of it draws additional attention to it. The patient's attempt to hide it by growing a long sideburn has failed. Retrodisplacement of bearded skin against the scar has resulted in a thin, spindly, unnatural, and unmasculine-appearing sideburn. (*B*) An unknown surgeon failed to recognize the difference in color and texture of the ear (tragal) and cheek skin and the use of a pretragal incision has resulted in an obvious irregularity even though the scar itself is well healed and difficult to see. The difference in color and texture on each side of the scar would be better concealed along anatomic interfaces if a retrotragal (see **Figs. 12–14**) incision plan had been used. Procedures performed by unknown surgeons. (*Courtesy of* Timothy Marten, MD, FACS, San Francisco, CA.)

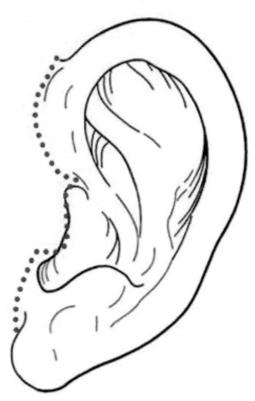

Fig. 12. Retrotragal plan for the preauricular portion of the facelift incision. Placing the incision along natural anatomic contours conceals the scar and disguises differences in color and skin texture on each side of it (see also **Figs. 13 and 14**). (*Courtesy of* Timothy Marten, MD, FACS, San Francisco, CA.)

anterior border of the helix and continued inferiorly, anterior to the tragus in a pretragal location (**Fig. 10**).

This plan, however, works well only for the unusual male patient with cheek and tragal skin of similar characteristics who, in addition, exhibits favorable healing. Unfortunately, most male patients have a marked gradient of color, texture, and surface irregularities over these areas and a telltale mismatch is evident, even in the presence of an inconspicuous scar (**Fig. 11**).

For these reasons, and in all but the unusual case, the preauricular portion of the facelift incision in men is usually best placed along the posterior margin of the tragus, rather than in the pretragal sulcus (**Figs. 12–14**).

In this location a mismatch of color, texture, or surface irregularities is not noticed and the scar, if visible, seems to be a tragal highlight (see **Fig. 13**).

In addition, if properly planned and executed, an incision along the margin of the tragus does not produce tragal retraction or other anatomic irregularity (see **Fig. 14**).

If tissue repositioning is achieved using SMAS advancement[9,10] and not excessive skin tension as it rightly should be, modest displacement of skin occurs in many male patients and no bearded skin is advanced onto the tragus (see **Fig. 14**A). In the male patient in whom large skin flap shifts occur, beard growth on the tragus is reduced by intraoperative destruction of beard follicles from the underside of the tragal flap (**Fig. 35**).

Because beard hair grows in three phases, beard shift encroachment on the tragus cannot usually be completely eliminated at the time of surgery. Most mature men in the facelift age group have some stray hair growth on the tragal area naturally, however, and some visible hair growth on the tragus is not necessarily seen as a sign a facelift has been performed in the eyes of most casual observers and in typical social situations (see **Fig. 7, 8, 13, 14**). To obtain the most natural appearance, some men may wish to undergo electrolysis following their surgery in the rare case that bearded skin is advanced onto the tragus and intraoperative epilation is not adequate. In general, it is prudent to wait 4 to 6 months after surgery before that is done.

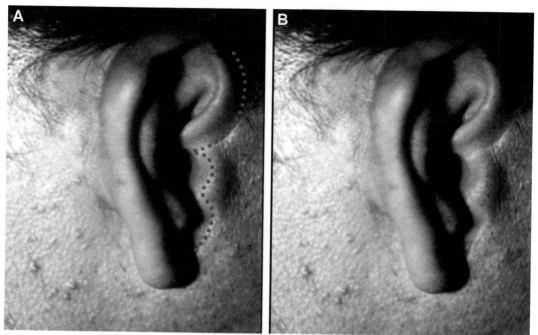

Fig. 13. Retrotragal incision plan and resulting scar. (*A*) Retrotragal plan for concealed preauricular incision (*dotted line*). The incision is planned along natural anatomic interfaces to disguise gradients of color and texture typically seen between the ear and cheek. (*B*) Healed retrotragal scar in a male facelift patient. The scar is situated along anatomic interfaces concealing gradients of color and texture that would be obvious if a pretragal incision plan had been used. In this location the scar if seen, fools the eye, and seems to be a reflected highlight. Procedure performed by Timothy Marten, MD, FACS. (*Courtesy of* Timothy Marten, MD, FACS, San Francisco, CA.)

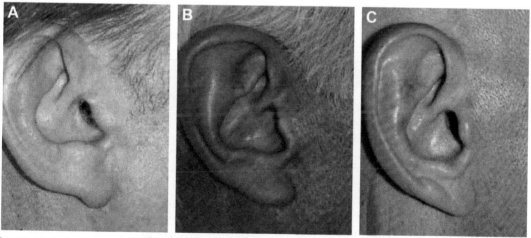

Fig. 14. Healed retrotragal facelift scars in male patients. (*A*) Retrotragal placement of the preauricular portion of the facelift incision has resulted in inconspicuous and well-concealed scars. In the upper third, the scar sits in the interface between the helix and the cheek and the scar seems to be a reflected highlight of the anterior helical border. In the middle third, the scar sits along the posterior margin of the tragus and cannot be seen. (*B* and *C*) Some coarse and bearded skin has been shifted up against and onto the tragus, but this is less obvious than the presence of a pretragal scar with a gradient of color and texture on each side of it. In the lower third, the scar sits in a well-concealed location 2 to 3 mm outside the lobular-facial sulcus but far enough away from it that shaving in that area is not difficult. All surgical procedures performed by Timothy Marten, MD, FACS. (*Courtesy of* Timothy Marten, MD, FACS, San Francisco, CA)

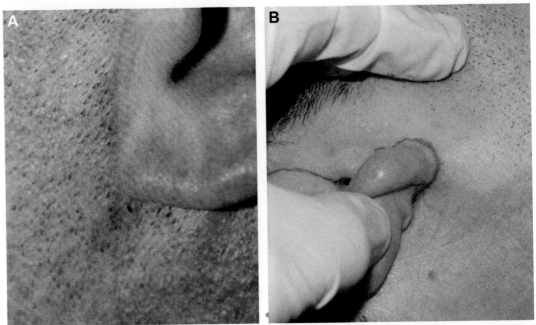

Fig. 15. Erroneous elimination of the lobular-facial sulcus and proper perilobular incision plan. (*A*) The perilobular incision has been placed too close to the earlobe and the lobular-facial sulcus eliminated. The thin, soft earlobe has been inserted into coarse, thick, bearded cheek skin resulting in an unnatural transition between the two structures and a facelifted appearance. Failure to preserve a cuff of lobular facial sulcus also makes it difficult for men to shave (procedure performed by unknown surgeon). (*B*) To obtain a natural perilobular appearance, and to facilitate shaving in men, it is prudent to mark the perilobular incision 2 to 3 mm inferior to the lobular-facial sulcus and slightly more inferior than it would be made a woman. All other factors being equal, a superior result is obtained when such a plan is used, in comparison with any plan where the incision is placed directly in the sulcus and an attempt is subsequently made to directly join thin, soft earlobe with coarse, thick cheek. (*Courtesy of* Timothy Marten, MD, FACS, San Francisco, CA)

The superior portion of the preauricular incision should be planned as a soft curve paralleling the curve of the anterior border of the helix. This results in a natural-appearing width to the helix in keeping with the rest of the ear and the resultant scar, if visible, appears to be a helical highlight. As the tragus is approached, the mark for incision is carried into the depression superior to it and

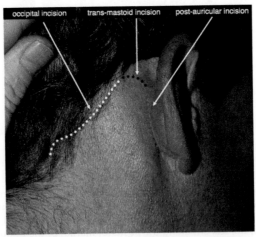

Fig. 16. Planning the postauricular incision. The postauricular incision (*red dotted line*) should be made 2 to 3 mm posterior to the existing auriculomastoid sulcus and the mark turned posteriorly to cross the mastoid at the approximate level of the anterior crus of the antihelix (see **Fig. 17**). Such a plan places the scar along a natural anatomic interface where it is difficult to detect but facilitates shaving of beard hair that might be advanced into this area. (*Courtesy of* Timothy Marten, MD, FACS, San Francisco, CA.)

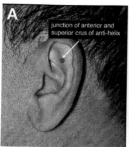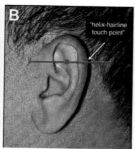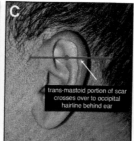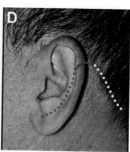

Fig. 17. Planning the position of the transmastoid part of the postauricular incision. Strategically placing the transmastoid part of the postauricular incision conceals it and allows optimal excision of skin from the anterior neck. If it is placed too low it is visible. If it is placed too high the defect created forces an overly vertical shift of the postauricular skin flap and compromises improvement in the neck. (*A*) The point of divergence of the anterior and superior crus of the helix provides a useful guide as to how high the transmastoid part of the postauricular incision should be placed (*red dot*). (*B*) At this horizontal level (*red line*) the rim of the helix typically touches the occipital hairline in the lateral view. (*C*) A transmastoid scar placed at this level crosses over to the occipital scalp in a hidden location. Note that if the incision were placed lower the resulting scar would show. (*D*) Typical plan for the postauricular incision showing the transmastoid component (*red line*) to be concealed (*gray dotted line* shows location of the auriculomastoid component incision hidden behind the ear and *white dotted line* the occipital incision hidden along the occipital hairline). Note that the male patient shown in **Fig. 17** has undergone a previous facelift and it is seen that his scars are well concealed despite his very short military style haircut. (Procedure performed by Timothy Marten MD). (*Courtesy of* Timothy Marten, MD, FACS, San Francisco, CA)

then continued along its posterior margin. In this location the scar, if visible, appears to be a natural highlight (see **Fig. 8, 12, 13, 14**).

At the inferior portion of the tragus the incision must turn anteriorly and then again inferiorly, into the crease between anterior lobule and cheek. If a more relaxed "lazy S" plan is made, or if a straight-line incision is used, skin settling and scar contraction result in crowding of the incisura, obliteration of the inferior tragal border, and a telltale elongated and chopped off and unnatural tragal appearance.

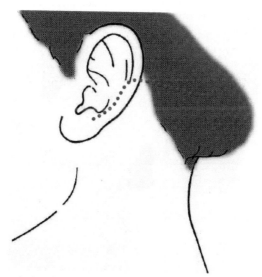

Fig. 18. Traditional (but incorrect) plan for the occipital portion of the facelift incision. In traditional facelift incision plans the incision is placed transversely on the occipital scalp in a well-intended but usually counterproductive attempt to hide the resultant scar. This incision plan does not allow for the excision of neck skin along an appropriate vector without resulting in notching and displacement of the occipital hairline (see **Fig. 19**) and is only applicable to young men with minimal neck skin excess who need little or no neck skin excised. (*Courtesy of* Timothy Marten, MD, FACS, San Francisco, CA)

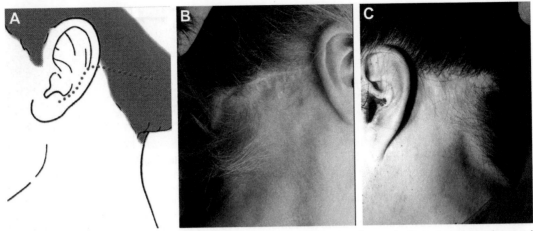

Fig. 19. Notching of the occipital hairline because of poor incision planning and attempts to hide the scar in scalp hair. (*A*) Traditional occipital incision plan responsible for notching of the hairline. (*B and C*) Examples of notching of the occipital hairline seen in two patients whose surgeons used traditional occipital incision plans that resulted in neck skin being advanced into areas where hair-bearing scalp should be present. Procedures performed by unknown surgeons. (*Courtesy of* Timothy Marten, MD, FACS, San Francisco, CA.)

Planning the perilobular incision

To obtain a natural perilobular appearance, and to facilitate shaving in men, it is essential whenever possible to preserve the natural sulcus of beard-free skin naturally present between the ear lobe and the cheek and to avoid destruction of, or excision of, this functionally and aesthetically important area when possible. This is accomplished by marking the perilobular incision 2 to 3 mm inferior to the lobular-facial sulcus and slightly lower than it would be made in a woman (**Fig. 15**B). All other factors being equal, a superior result is obtained

when such a plan is used, in comparison with any plan where the incision is placed directly in the sulcus and an attempt is subsequently made to directly join thin, soft earlobe with coarse, thick bearded cheek skin (**Fig. 15**A). Preserving the lobular-facial sulcus also makes it significantly easier for the patient to shave in the perilobular area.

Planning the postauricular incision

Traditionally, the postauricular portion of the face-lift incision has been made in men and women up

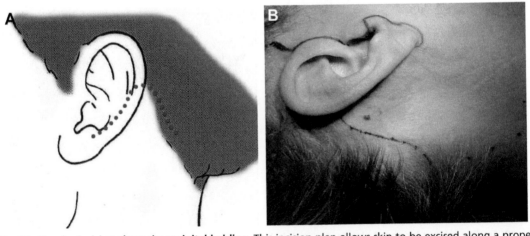

Fig. 20. Plan for incision along the occipital hairline. This incision plan allows skin to be excised along a proper posterior-superior vector, prevents hairline displacement, and results in a well-concealed scar if carried out in a technically correct fashion. Note that the incision is planned so that its inferior portion typically turns posteriorly into the occipital scalp at the junction of thick and thin hair but varies in length in accord with the amount of skin redundancy present in the anterior neck area (see **Fig. 21**). (*A*) Schematic of occipital hairline incision plan. (*B*) Occipital hairline incision plan marked on a patient. (*Courtesy of* Timothy Marten, MD, FACS, San Francisco, CA.)

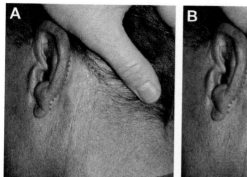
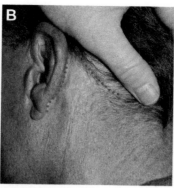
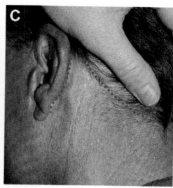

Fig. 21. Plan for length of incision along the occipital hairline. The length of the occipital portion of the postauricular incision (*red dotted line*) varies depending on the quality of the patient's tissues and the amount of redundant skin present in the submental area (size of the wattle). (*A*) In patients with good tissue quality and minimal submental skin redundancy (small wattle) a short incision along the hairline is indicated. (*B*) In patients with modest loss of skin quality and modest submental redundancy (medium wattle) a medium incision is made along the occipital hairline. (*C*) In elderly patients with poor skin elasticity and a large submental skin excess (large wattle) a long incision along the occipital hairline is needed. (*Courtesy of* Timothy Marten, MD, FACS, San Francisco, CA.)

over the posterior surface of the concha. This was done as part of a well-intended effort to offset inevitable descent of the postauricular flap and inferior migration of the resulting scar that occurred when skin was tightened in a misguided attempt to improve neck contour. Many surgeons have come to realize that such a plan embodies several erroneous assumptions and can result in undesirable and problematic effects including hypertrophic scarring, postauricular webbing, and obliteration of the auriculomastoid sulcus. If such a plan is used in men, bearded skin from the neck can also be moved up into the auriculomastoid sulcus, or even onto the posterior surface of the ear resulting in considerable difficulty in shaving.

The postauricular portion of the facelift incision in the male patient should instead be marked 2

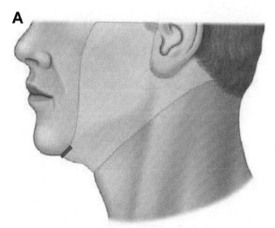
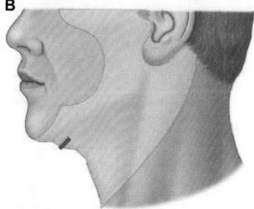

Fig. 22. Planning the submental incision. (*A*) Traditional, but incorrect plan for the submental incision (*red line*) and skin undermining. The incision should not be placed directly along the submental crease because this accentuates it and reinforces the double chin appearance. Note that typical plan of skin undermining (*yellow shaded area*) also promotes a double chin because the crease is not undermined, retaining ligaments are not released, and fat of the chin and submental region cannot be blended. (*B*) Correct location for the submental incision (*red line*). Placing the submental incision posterior to the submental crease prevents accentuation of the double chin appearance and provides for easier dissection and suturing in the anterior neck (compare with **Fig. 22**A). Note that this incision plan allows the submental crease to be undermined (*yellow shaded area*), the submental restraining ligaments to be released, and the fat of the chin pad and neck to be blended.

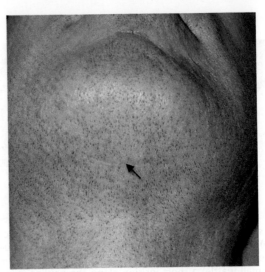

Fig. 23. **Healed submental incision in a male patient.** Placement of the submental incision posterior to the submental crease still results in an inconspicuous, well-concealed scar and allows the submental crease to be released and the double chin to be corrected. The submental incision should be made precisely parallel to beard follicles to minimize injury to them. Procedure performed by Timothy Marten, MD, FACS. (*Courtesy of* Timothy Marten, MD, FACS, San Francisco, CA.)

to 3 mm posterior to the existing auriculomastoid sulcus with the ear pulled forward as little as possible, and the mark turned posteriorly to cross the mastoid at the approximate level of the anterior crus of the antihelix. Such a plan places the scar at a natural anatomic interface where it is difficult to detect, even on close inspection (**Fig. 2**; **Fig. 16**) but facilitates shaving of beard hair that might be advanced onto this area.

Planning the transmastoid portion of the postauricular incision

Considerable confusion exists among surgeons performing facelift procedures as to what level the transmastoid part of the postauricular facelift incision (see **Fig. 16** black dotted line) should cross over to the occipital scalp and as a result this part of the incision is often not placed strategically and in a manner that best conceals it, or in a

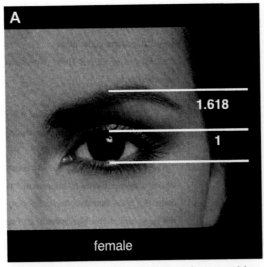

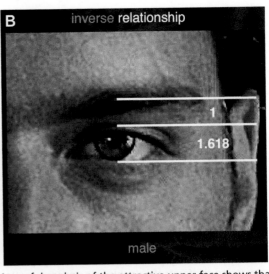

Fig. 24. **The golden proportion and eyebrow position.** A careful analysis of the attractive upper face shows that the aperture of the eye (the vertical distance between the upper and lower eyelids in forward gaze) and the distance between the margin of the upper lid and arch of the eyebrow is described by the golden proportion. It is a commonly observed fact that male and female eyebrow positions are not the same and intuitively obvious that eyebrow position connotes sex differences. (*A*) The "golden eyebrow" in a woman. (*B*) The "golden eyebrow" in a man. For most men the attractive eyebrow falls in inverse relation to that of the female but remains in golden proportion to the palpebral aperture. (*Courtesy of* Timothy Marten, MD, FACS, San Francisco, CA.)

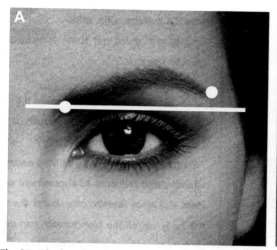
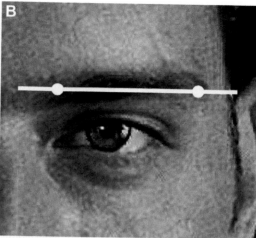

Fig. 25. Ideal eyebrow shape in women and men. (*A*) The female brow appears attractive at a variety of heights if it is in an arched configuration with its tail higher than its medial aspect (*white dots* represent position of medial and lateral aspects of the eyebrow; *white line* shows horizontal). (*B*) The male brow appears attractive at a variety of heights if it is in a near horizontal configuration with its tail at the same height as its medial aspect, or slightly superior to it. (*Courtesy of* Timothy Marten, MD, FACS, San Francisco, CA.)

way that allows optimal excision of skin from the anterior neck. If it is placed too low it is visible in the male patient who typically wears a short hairstyle. If it is placed too high the defect created forces an overly vertical shift of the postauricular skin flap and compromises improvement in the anterior neck and submental region.

A useful guide in siting the transmastoid part of the postauricular incision is to envision a horizontal line through the point at which the anterior and superior crus of the antihelix diverge (red dot in **Fig. 17**A). Typically at that level the rim of the helix extends posteriorly back to the occipital hairline to the so-called "helix-hairline touch point" (**Fig. 17**B) and a transmastoid incision placed at that level is hidden behind the ear in the lateral view (see **Fig. 17**C, D).

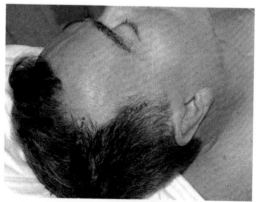

Fig. 26. Small incision temple and forehead lift. Most men need conservative treatment of their forehead and brow and many are well served with a sort scar small incision plan as shown. The incision on the temporal scalp is used to make a subgaleal dissection and the incision on the parietal scalp is used to make a subperiosteal dissection. A lateral forehead flap is mobilized by subsequently releasing the temporal line of adherence and dividing the periosteum under the lateral aspect of the eyebrow. An endoscope is not always necessarily required and the latter maneuvers can often be accomplished under direct vision through the incision on the temporal scalp. (*Courtesy of* Timothy Marten, MD, FACS, San Francisco, CA.)

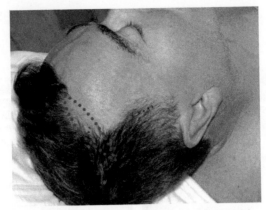

Fig. 27. Partial hairline forehead-temple lift incision plan. Partial hairline incisions are useful in some men as a means of reducing temporal hairline recession and reducing forehead redundancy. This plan should result in an inconspicuous scar if the incisions are meticulously closed under no tension. (*Courtesy of* Timothy Marten, MD, FACS, San Francisco, CA.)

Planning the occipital incision

Planning the location for the occipital portion of the facelift incision is conceptually similar to that of the temple region and the incision plan must address similar concerns of hairline displacement and scar visibility. Traditionally this incision is placed transversely extending into the occipital scalp in men and women, in a well-intended but usually counterproductive attempt to hide the resultant scar (**Fig. 18**).

For patients in whom neck skin redundancy is small and excision of postauricular skin is unnecessary, such a plan may be acceptable and results in a well-concealed scar. Male patients in this category are usually young and troubled by mild

neck deformity only, and in these situations the incision is used for access to the lateral neck only, and not as a means to remove postauricular skin. Mistakenly using this incision plan to excise skin predictably results in the advancement of neck skin into the occipital scalp and notching of the occipital hairline (**Fig. 19**).

Although women sometimes can hide such a deformity because of the presence of longer hair, creating a step-off and hairline displacement on a male patient can result in a problem that is difficult to conceal and correct.

Proper analysis, careful planning, and the use of an incision along the hairline (**Fig. 20**), when indicated and carried out in a technically correct

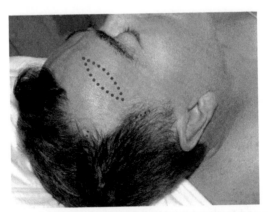

Fig. 28. Forehead crease temple-forehead lift incision plan. Bald or balding men, men who wear very short hairstyles, men who have previously had hair transplants and fear disruption of their hairline, and men with shaved heads are effectively treated using an incision in a horizontal forehead crease. Skin only is excised and minimum undermining only is usually required. The scar once healed is often less conspicuous than the forehead crease it was planned around. This plan allows lifting of the temporal face and the eyebrow, and reduction of temporal redundancy that is sometimes generated by a facelift procedure. (*Courtesy of* Timothy Marten, MD, FACS, San Francisco, CA.)

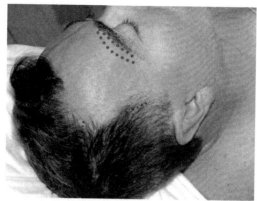

Fig. 29. Superciliary direct eyebrow lift incision plan. Bald or balding men, men who wear very short hairstyles, men who have previously had hair transplants and fear disruption of their hairline, and men with shaved heads are effectively treated using an incision along the upper margin of the eyebrow. Skin only is excised and minimum undermining only is usually required. The scar once healed is typically inconspicuous, especially in men in the facelift age group. This plan does not allow lifting of the temporal face and is not helpful in reducing temporal redundancy that is sometimes generated by a facelift procedure. (*Courtesy of* Timothy Marten, MD, FACS, San Francisco, CA.)

manner, prevents this problem and allows skin to be excised along a correct posterior-superior vector, while simultaneously producing a well-concealed scar (see **Fig. 2**).

The length of the occipital portion of the post-auricular incision necessarily varies depending on the quality of the patient's tissues and the amount of redundant skin present in the anterior neck and

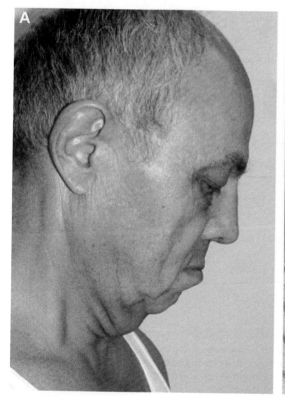
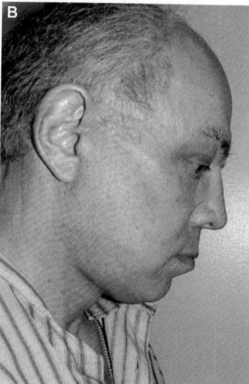

Fig. 30. The neck comprises a key element of rejuvenating the male face. Neck improvement is of high priority to almost every male patient seeking facial rejuvenation, and the results of male facelift procedures are often largely judged by the outcome achieved in the neck. (*A*) Preoperative view of male patient with poor neckline. (*B*) After view of same patient. A more fit, athletic, masculine, and decisive appearance is seen. All surgical procedures performed by Timothy Marten, MD, FACS. (*Courtesy of* Timothy Marten, MD, FACS, San Francisco, CA.)

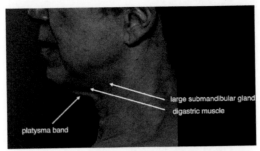

Fig. 31. Deep layer neck problems. The patient has undergone a previous facelift and neck lift performed by an unknown surgeon in which submental liposuction and tightening of neck skin was performed. It is seen that although the submental area has been stripped of subcutaneous fat this approach ignored several anatomic problems present in most males including platysmal laxity, platysma bands, excess subplatysmal fat, large submandibular glands, and digastric muscle hypertrophy. Removing subcutaneous fat and tightening skin over these problems does not correct them. (*Courtesy of* Timothy Marten, MD, FACS, San Francisco, CA.)

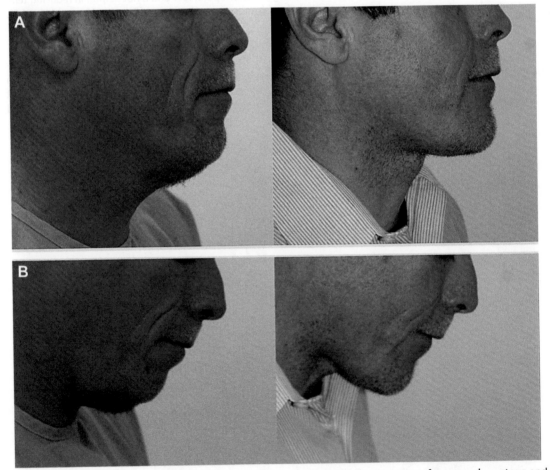

Fig. 32. Treating the chin in the male patient. The difference between the presence of poor neck contour and microgenia is commonly misunderstood, and it is a common misconception that placement of a chin implant improves neck contour. Placement of a chin implant when microgenia is not present is a conceptual and artistic error that creates unnatural appearances. (*A*) Patient seen preoperatively has poor neck contour made worse by the presence of mild to moderate microgenia. (*B*) Same patient following short scar neck lift and chin implant placement (a submental incision only was made and the patient has no scar around the ears). When true microgenia is present placing a chin implant in combination with a neck lift produces a more a more aesthetic, athletic, and attractive cervicofacial relationship. The patient has not only better neck contour, but a more harmonious and balanced profile. All surgical procedures performed by Timothy Marten, MD, FACS. (*Courtesy of* Timothy Marten, MD, FACS, San Francisco, CA.)

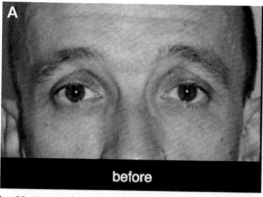 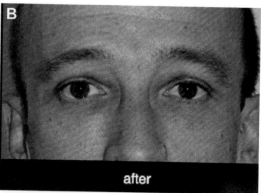

Fig. 33. Fat grafting the upper orbit. Atrophy often plays a far greater role in the changes seen in the male orbital area with age than is appreciated, and replenishing lost orbital fat is profoundly rejuvenating in male patients. Traditional blepharoplasty in these patients actually degrades the appearance of the eye. (*A*) Patient seen preoperatively with hollow upper orbits. He has an aged and unmasculine appearance. (*B*) Same patient after periorbital fat grafting. The patient has a younger, more fit, healthy, attractive, and masculine appearance (patient has also undergone fat grafting to his temples, radix, cheeks, and midface). All surgical procedures performed by Timothy Marten, MD, FACS. (*Courtesy of* Timothy Marten, MD, FACS, San Francisco, CA.)

submental area (size of wattle), and small, medium, and long (length of incision along the occipital hairline) incision plans are used as indicated (**Fig. 21**). In patients with good tissue quality and minimal anterior neck and submental skin excess (small wattle) a short incision along the hairline is indicated (see **Fig. 21**A). In patients with modest loss of skin quality and modest anterior neck and submental skin excess (medium wattle) a medium-length incision is made along the occipital hairline (see **Fig. 21**B). In elderly patients with poor skin elasticity and a large anterior neck and submental skin excess (large wattle) a long incision along the occipital hairline is needed (see **Fig. 21**C).

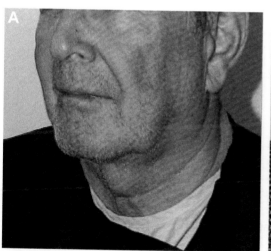 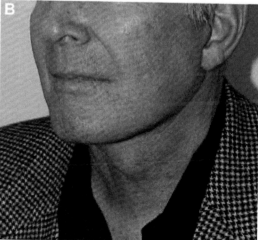

Fig. 34. Strengthening the male jawline using fat grafting. The young attractive, athletic, and masculine face is characterized a rectangular shape and a strong mandibular contour. Replenishing lost volume along the mandible restores a more youthful male facial shape and a more bold and decisive appearance. (*A*) Patient seen preoperatively. The posterior jawline is weak and an indistinct transition from the face to the neck is present. (*B*) The same patient after a facelift and neck lift that included fat grafting. Fat grafting has been used to strengthen the cheek and jawline and create a more bold, athletic, youthful, and masculine mandibular contour. A distinct transition from the cheek to the neck is now present. No facial implants were placed. All surgical procedures performed by Timothy Marten, MD, FACS. (Courtesy of Timothy Marten, MD, FACS, San Francisco, CA.)

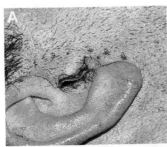 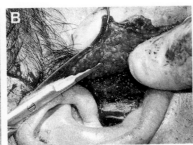 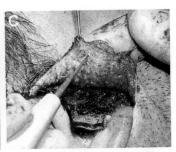

Fig. 35. Epilation of beard follicles from tragus. In the older male patient in whom large skin flap shifts occur, beard growth on the tragus is reduced by intraoperative destruction of beard follicles from the underside of the skin flap. (*A*) The facelift flap has been trimmed but has not been sutured. Beard hair has been shifted into a normally non-hair-bearing area (area posterior to *purple dotted line*). Note patient has not shaved for 2 days preoperatively. (*B*) The preauricular skin flap is inverted over the surgeon's fingertip using small skin hook retractors. Because the patient has not shaved for several days preoperatively, beard stubble pushes the beard follicles out of the plane of the skin on the underside of the flap. Excising subcutaneous fat as shown further exposes the unwanted beard follicles and results in the direct removal of some follicles. (*C*) Using loupe magnification and a needle-tipped cautery set on a very low setting, remaining follicles and residual follicle elements are epilated. Care must be taken to only cauterize follicles and not apply cautery current to the skin itself. (*Courtesy of* Timothy Marten, MD, FACS, San Francisco, CA.)

Planning the submental incision

Optimal improvement in the neck can generally not be obtained in most male patients unless a submental incision is made because of the near universal presence of excess subplatysmal fat, large submandibular glands, and hypertrophy and/or malposition of the anterior bellies of the digastric muscles typically seen in most men presenting for facelift surgery. Simply performing liposuction, suspending the lateral platysma border, and/or tightening skin over these problems (**Fig. 31**) cannot correct them or produce the type of necklines associated with a fit, athletic, youthful, and healthy-appearing man **Figs 3, 4, 30, 37-39, 40–43, and 44–48**.

Traditionally the submental incision in male patients has been placed directly in and along the submental crease in a well-intended but practically counterproductive attempt to conceal the resulting scar (**Fig. 22A**).

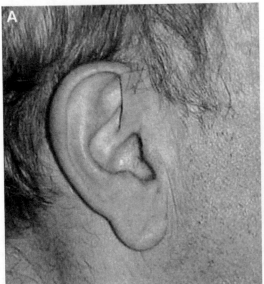 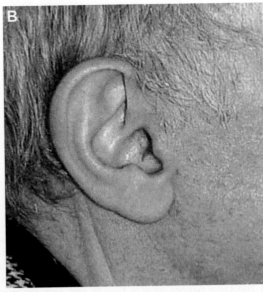

Fig. 36. Earlobe reduction. (*A*) Preoperative close-up view of male ear. The large earlobe lends the patients a telltale old and aged "grandfatherly" appearance. (*B*) Same patient after a facelift that included earlobe reduction. The ear appears, smaller, younger, and more proportionate. All surgical procedures performed by Timothy Marten, MD, FACS. (*Courtesy of* Timothy Marten, MD, FACS, San Francisco, CA.)

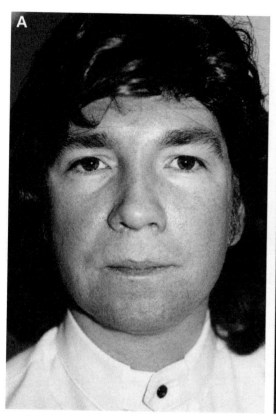 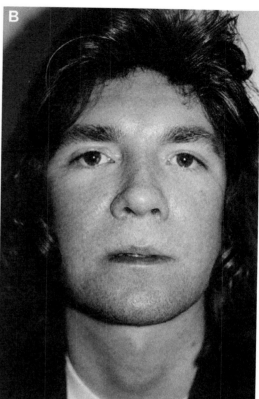

Fig. 37. Patient example 1 (front view). (*A*) Before surgery view of patient, age 42. The patient has full upper eyelids, ptotic, hollow upper cheeks, deep cheek folds, and a weak-appearing jawline. (*B*) Same patient, 2 years and 3 months after facelift, neck lift, small incision forehead lift, upper and lower eye lifts, fat grafting, and chin implant. Note corrections of hooded eyelids, diminished cheek folds, and creation of a youthful and masculine facial shape without a tight or pulled appearance. All surgical procedures performed by Timothy Marten, MD, FACS. (*Courtesy of* Timothy Marten, MD, FACS, San Francisco, CA.)

This incision plan should be avoided, however, because it surgically reinforces the crease and accentuates a double chin appearance. Exposure of the submental region is also compromised, and difficulty is encountered when dissecting, performing deep layer neck maneuvers, and when suturing low in the neck. A more posterior placement of this incision eliminates these problems, but still results in an inconspicuous and well-concealed scar (**Figs. 22B and 23**).

The submental incision should be placed well within the mandibular shadow and well posterior but parallel to the submental crease at a point lying roughly one-half the distance between the mentum and hyoid. This usually corresponds to a site situated 1.5 to 2 cm posterior to the crease. The incision should be approximately 3.5 cm in length, but may be made longer as long as neither end is advanced up on a visible portion of the face when cheek skin flaps are shifted. Healing is best, and the scar are best concealed, if it is made as a

straight, and not as a curved line, precisely parallel to beard hair shafts and beard follicles (see **Fig. 23**). Skin should never be excised from the submental crease.

Treating the Forehead in the Male Facelift Patient

One of the most frequent errors made by plastic surgeons in treating the male patient is performing upper blepharoplasty when a foreheadplasty is needed. As the forehead ages the brow descends and infrabrow skin moves into the upper orbit producing an illusion of eyelid skin redundancy. This false excess of upper eyelid skin is known as "pseudodermatochalasis," a term that emphasizes the deceptive origin of the problem and one that rightly draws attention to the need to consider forehead surgery in its treatment.

Attempts to treat pseudodermatochalasis with blepharoplasty alone at best result in a sad,

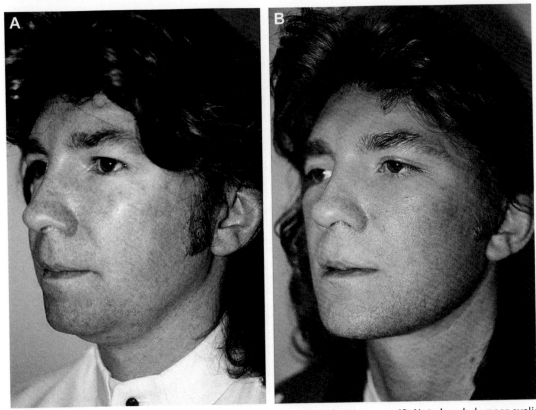

Fig. 38. Patient example 1 (oblique view). (*A*) Before surgery view of patient age 42. Note hooded upper eyelid, sagging cheek, hollow lower orbit, and loss of youthful neck and jawline contour. (*B*) Same patient, 2 years and 3 months after facelift, neck lift, closed forehead lift, upper and lower eye lifts, fat grafting, and chin implant. Note softer appearance to eyes, improved cheek contours, masculine jawline, and improved neck contour. The chin contour is also improved and the patient has a rested, fit, athletic, decisive, and masculine appearance. All surgical procedures performed by Timothy Marten, MD, FACS. (*Courtesy of* Timothy Marten, MD, FACS, San Francisco, CA.)

tired-appearing patient, poor eyebrow position and configuration, less eyelid skin, and a long scar extending off the eyelid and well onto the lateral periorbital/temporal skin. More likely, however, isolated blepharoplasty performed when significant forehead/eyebrow ptosis is present usually results in a loss of the stimulus for brow elevation, further descent of the eyebrow as the frontalis muscle relaxes, and the reappearance of a pseudoskin excess in the superior-lateral orbit and across the upper eyelid as infrabrow skin moves into the orbit. This, in turn, results in an exacerbation of the existing pseudosad, pseudo-tired, or disinterested appearance, rather than improvement in it. This sequence of events explains why many male patients and their surgeons are often disappointed with the patient's overall appearance after upper blepharoplasty, despite technical proficiency in the excision of upper eyelid tissue.

A key requirement in planning rejuvenation of the male forehead when it is indicated is understanding male brow aesthetics and optimal position and configuration of the male eyebrow. Proper position and configuration of the eyebrow is ultimately a subjective judgment in all patients influenced by racial, cultural, and other factors that cannot be determined precisely by a fixed mathematical formula or arbitrary measurement, and marks, measurements, and published parameters should be regarded as guidelines in planning surgery. These are not appropriate in every situation or absolutely correct for every face. Ultimately, and as in the female face, the artistic imperative is to achieve proportion and balance with other facial features.[15,18]

Traditionally, surgeons have tried to define ideal eyebrow position in simple linear and absolute terms. Although convenient, and useful to some extent, any such analysis is intrinsically flawed in that rigid linear measurements are ultimately

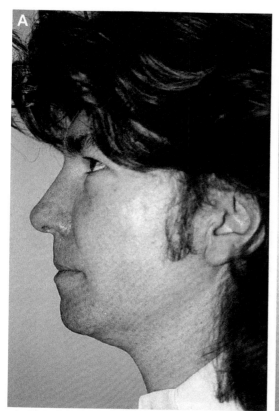
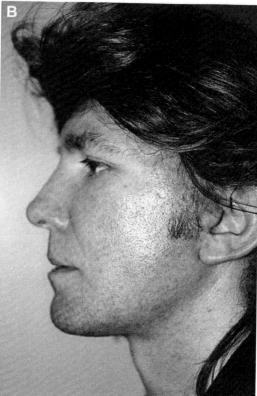

Fig. 39. Patient example 1 (side view). (*A*) Before surgery view of patient age 42. Note lower eyelid fullness, poor transition from the lower eyelid to the cheek, poor jawline, weak chin, and full neck. (*B*) Same patient, 2 years and 3 months after facelift, neck lift, closed forehead lift, upper and lower eye lifts, fat grafting, and chin implant. The transition from the lower eyelid to the cheek is smoother; the cheek position has been improved; chin contour is improved; and a fit, athletic, masculine-appearing jawline and neckline is seen. The face has a natural appearance and all scars are well concealed. All surgical procedures performed by Timothy Marten, MD, FACS. (*Courtesy of* Timothy Marten, MD, FACS, San Francisco, CA.)

inaccurate in that they assume each subject's head and facial features to be the same size. A more accurate and appropriate guide to what is appropriate and attractive is the "golden proportion." Simply stated, the golden proportion specifies that when the proportions of a facial feature, or relationship between two facial features, are described by a ratio of 1 to 1.618, they appear attractive and pleasing to the eye.

A careful analysis of the attractive upper face shows that the aperture of the eye (the vertical distance between the upper and lower eyelids in forward gaze) and the distance between the margin of the upper lid and arch of the eyebrow are related to one another by the golden proportion.

It is a commonly observed fact that male and female eyebrow positions are not the same and intuitively obvious that eyebrow position connotes sex differences. For most men, however, the attractive eyebrow falls in inverse relationship to that of the female but remains in golden proportion to the palpebral aperture (**Fig. 24**).

Although more useful than any arbitrary fixed linear distance, the golden proportion should also be recognized as a guideline to eyebrow position and not an absolute ideal, and that under certain circumstances a higher or lower position may be regarded as appropriate and attractive. Perhaps the most useful clinical guideline is simply that the male brow is generally regarded as attractive at a variety of heights if it is in a horizontal or near horizontal configuration with its tail at the same height as its medial aspect, or slightly superior to it (**Fig. 25**). Said differently, the goal is not so much to lift the eyebrow higher as it is to tilt it and shape it, and if one can achieve good eyebrow shape most patients and their surgeons are happy.

There are several useful forehead lift strategies applicable to the male patient and there is no one procedure that is appropriate for all patients.

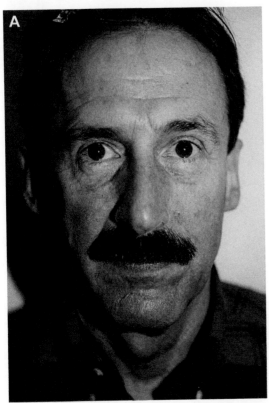
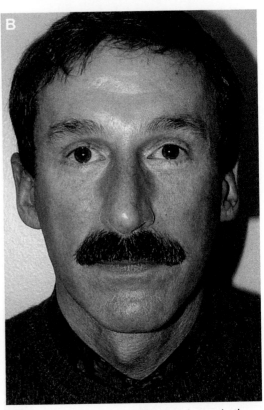

Fig. 40. Patient example 2 (front view). (*A*) Before surgery view of patient, age 60. Hollowness is seen in the under eye and upper cheek area. Loss of youthful facial contour is seen in the cheek and jowl areas. (*B*) Same patient, 1 year 2 months after facelift, neck lift, small incision forehead lift, upper and lower eye lifts, and partial facial fat transfer. Fat injections have provided filling of the under eye and cheek areas. Note restoration of youthful facial shape without a tight or pulled appearance. All surgical procedures performed by Timothy Marten, MD, FACS. (*Courtesy of* Timothy Marten, MD, FACS, San Francisco, CA.)

Coronal and hairline incision forehead lifts are only occasionally indicated in the male patient, and most male patients' objectives are met by simpler strategies that do not sacrifice hair including small incision, partial hairline, forehead crease, and superciliary direct eyebrow lifts.

Small incision lifts are possible in men with receding hairlines and the bald or balding man if incisions are carefully sited (**Fig. 26** see also Case 1–3). Often, these lifts are much more technically difficult to carry out in men than in women, however, because of the thick, heavy forehead tissues typically present in men, and the greater distance at which one is working because of retrodisplaced, receded hairlines.

Partial hairline incisions are useful in some men as a means of reducing temporal hairline recession and actually reducing forehead redundancy, and should result in an inconspicuous scar if the wounds are closed carefully and under no tension. Typically these procedures are performed in a dual plane, subcutaneously in the lateral forehead and in a subgaleal place beneath the scalp. In most

men, hairline position and hair density are mostly stable by the time they reach facelift age, and concerns that hair might recede from the scar are largely unwarranted. This plan (see **Fig. 27**) may be off-putting to some men, however, who wear shorter hairstyles, have had hair transplants, or who are otherwise concerned with the visibility of the scar, but is highly effective if planned and carried out carefully.

Bald or balding men, men who wear very short hairstyles, men who have previously had hair transplants and fear disruption of their hairline, and men with shaved heads are effectively treated using an incision in a horizontal forehead crease (see **Fig. 28**) or in a superciliary direct eyebrow lift location along the superior margin of the eyebrow (see **Fig. 29**).

The superciliary direct eyebrow lift is particularly useful and well aligned with the needs of the older male with significant eyebrow ptosis who is resistant to a more complicated procedure using incisions along the hairline or within the scalp.

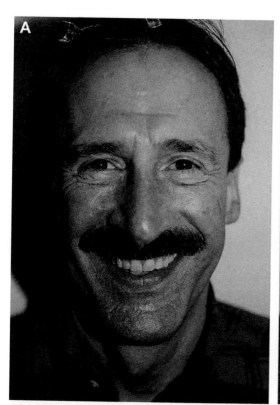
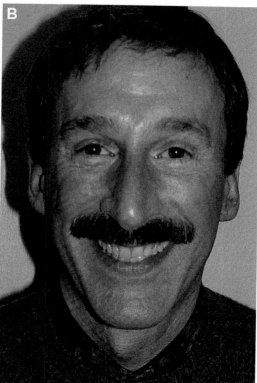

Fig. 41. Patient example 2 (front smiling view). (*A*) Before surgery view of patient, age 60. (*B*) Same patient, 1 year 2 months after facelift, neck lift, closed forehead lift, upper and lower eye lifts, and partial facial fat grafting. Note a natural appearance is present, even when smiling. All surgical procedures performed by Timothy Marten, MD, FACS. *Courtesy of* Timothy Marten, MD, FACS, San Francisco, CA

Treating the Neck in the Male Facelift Patient

A well-contoured neck is an artistic imperative to an attractive and appealing masculine appearance, and a bold, well-defined neckline conveys a sense of youth, health, fitness, strength, vitality, and decisiveness (**Fig. 30**). Neck improvement is of high priority to almost every male patient seeking facial rejuvenation, and the results of male facelift procedures are often largely judged by the outcome achieved in the neck. If the neck is not sufficiently improved, most male patients believe we have failed them.

Although it is a common strategy, it is not enough to perform submental liposuction and tighten the skin in most patients because such an approach ignores several anatomic problems present in most male patients seeking neck improvement including platysmal laxity; platysma bands; excess subplatysmal fat; large submandibular glands; digastric muscle hypertrophy; and developmental factors, such as the size and shape of the bony jaw and chin. Removing subcutaneous fat and tightening skin over these problems does not correct them, and the presence or absence

of each must be looked for to create an appropriate surgical plan (see **Fig. 31**).

Large anterior neck Z-plasties have been put forth as a means for direct treatment of the male neck by surgeons who have failed to meet their patients' needs with submental liposuction, and other conceptually flawed schemes. In some cases some surgeons combine anterior neck Z-plasties with subplatysmal fat reduction and "corset" platysma muscle suturing. In either case a large and objectionable-appearing anterior neck scar is created that is often hypertrophic, and Z-plasty flap transposition results in abnormally directed beard growth. Both of these occurrences are often troublesome for male patients. It is far more productive to treat deep layer neck problems in the male patient through a far smaller and better concealed submental incision (see **Figs. 22 and 23**), and to remove excess skin against the occipital hairline where the scar is far better concealed when indicated. The results that are obtained with short scar neck lift (see **Figs. 3 and 4**) make clear the relative unimportance of skin excision and lateral platysmal tightening.

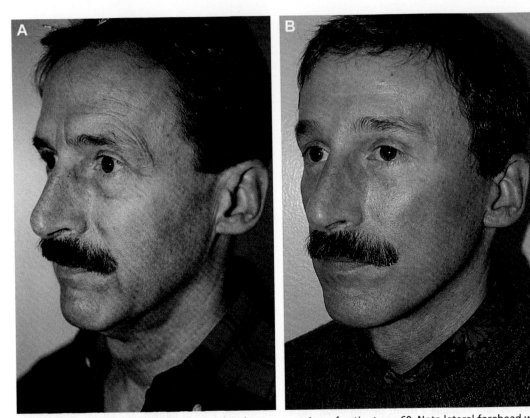

Fig. 42. Patient example 2 (oblique view). (*A*) Before surgery view of patient age 60. Note lateral forehead wrinkling, sagging cheek, and loss of youthful jawline contour. (*B*) Same patient, 1 year 2 months after facelift, neck lift, closed forehead lift, upper and lower eye lifts, and partial facial fat grafting. Note smoother forehead, restoration of cheek fullness, improved transition from lower lid to cheek, smooth, stronger jawline, and improved neck contour. All surgical procedures performed by Timothy Marten, MD, FACS. (*Courtesy of* Timothy Marten, MD, FACS, San Francisco, CA.)

Treating the Chin in the Male Facelift Patient

The difference between the presence of poor neck contour and microgenia is commonly misunderstood, and it is a common misconception that placement of a chin implant improves neck contour. A chin implant is a treatment for microgenia (not a poor neckline) and the presence or absence of microgenia and the need for a chin implant is a cephalometric determination that is independent of the condition of the neck. Placement of a chin implant when microgenia is not present is a conceptual and artistic error that creates unnatural appearances.

When true microgenia is present, however, placing a chin implant in combination with a neck lift produces a more harmonious and balanced profile, a more aesthetic and attractive cervicofacial relationship, and a bolder more athletic masculine appearance (**Fig. 32**, see also **Figs. 37–39**).

The male chin differs considerably from that of the female and the surgeon treating male patients must keep this in mind when planning and performing procedures. The male chin is broader, stronger, squarer, and has more vertical height than that of the female, and a strong chin and balanced profile are arguably more important to male attractiveness than to female beauty. A man with a weak chin typically is regarded as weak and indecisive appearing, and in some cases, even unmasculine and effeminate. The male chin should also be smoothly confluent and well-integrated with the jawline, with a smooth and seamless transition across the geniomandibular confluence (**Fig. 34** and **Figs. 37–39**).

Some strengthening of the male chin can be accomplished with fat grafting and fat grafting provides a means to readily increase vertical chin height. Often a chin implant is used together with fat grafting to optimize lower facial contour in the male patient, with the chin implant providing a reliable increase in chin projection and the fat used to

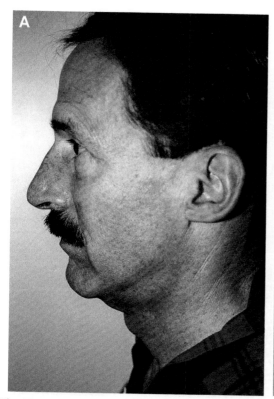 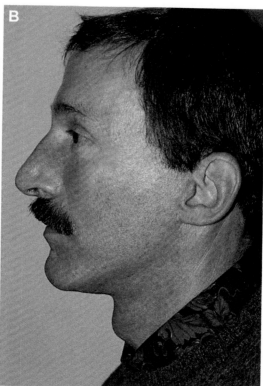

Fig. 43. Patient example 2 (side view). (*A*) Before surgery view of patient age 60. Note cheek flatness, sagging jawline, and neck laxity. A protruding salivary gland can also be seen in the neck area. (*B*) Same patient, 1 year 2 months after facelift, neck lift, forehead lift, upper and lower eye lift, and partial facial fat grafting. The protruding portion of the salivary gland has also been removed. Note the restoration of cheek fullness, smooth jawline, and improved neck contour. The face has a natural appearance and all scars are well concealed. All surgical procedures performed by Timothy Marten, MD, FACS. *Courtesy of* Timothy Marten, MD, FACS, San Francisco, CA

increase vertical height, fill the geniomandibular groove, and to avoid an overly deep and unnatural labiomental sulcus.

Eyelid Surgery in the Male Facelift Patient

The attractive male orbit and eyelid is distinctly full and however well intended, traditional blepharoplasty procedures in which eyelid skin and fat are aggressively removed can degrade the appearance of the male eye and result in an overly changed appearance in men.

Brow ptosis is often marked in many men and simply looking at and then treating the upper eyelid can result in inappropriate overexcision of eyelid skin and functional and aesthetic problems. For many men subtly repositioning the lateral brow and fixing it in the position the patient holds it as a result of frontalis muscle contraction, lifts the upper lid skin fold off the eyelashes and precludes the need for potentially functionally inappropriate

upper eyelid surgery that aesthetically degrades the appearance of the eye. When upper eyelid surgery is performed in men, it should be done conservatively. It is far better to perform a second-stage skin excision at some future date, than to remove too much skin at the primary procedure and create an overly changed, hollow, unmasculine, or ill appearance.

As is the case with many women, atrophy often plays a far greater role in the changes seen in the male orbital area with age, and replenishing lost orbital fat is profoundly rejuvenating in male patients (**Fig. 33**).

The typical male facelift patient often expresses concern about his lower eyelids but lower blepharoplasty, if indicated, must be performed cautiously because of the predictable presence of lower lid laxity in men. If the lower lid distracts more that 5 to 6 mm, which is common, some form of canthopexy is likely indicated if lid retraction and a sad, melancholic, aged appearance

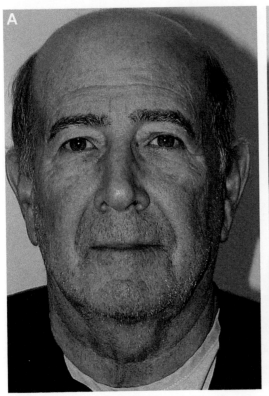
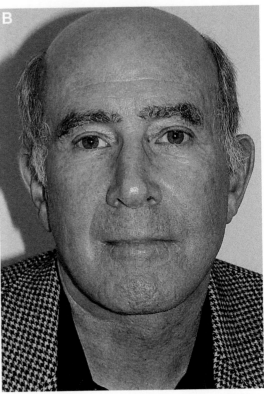

Fig. 44. Patient example 3 (front view). (*A*) Before surgery view of patient, age 68. The patient has eyebrow ptosis, full upper eyelids, sagging cheeks, deep cheek folds, and jowls. Loss of youthful facial contour is seen in the cheek and jowl areas. (*B*) Same patient, 1 year and 9 months after facelift, neck lift, small incision forehead lift, upper and lower eye lifts, partial facial fat grafting, and ear lobe reduction. Note improved eyebrow position and configuration, corrections of hooded eyelids, diminished cheek folds, elimination of jowls, and restoration of youthful and masculine facial shape without a tight or pulled appearance. All surgical procedures performed by Timothy Marten, MD, FACS. (*Courtesy of* Timothy Marten, MD, FACS, San Francisco, CA.)

(and potentially dry eye problems) are to be avoided.

Often what seems to be a large lower eyelid "bag" is in reality merely a pseudoherniation of orbital fat and in truth largely an atrophic midface and cheek. As such, replenishing lost midface and upper cheek volume is often more appropriate in those situations than removal of the lower eyelid "bag."

A good strategy that is commonly used in treating the eyelids in men undergoing facelift surgery, especially if they are public figures or are worried about an overly changed appearance, is to not perform traditional blepharoplasties as part of the procedure. Leaving the upper eyelid redundant, and a bag in the lower orbital area, preserves the patient's appearance in important loci of identity, and can dissuade others from believing any surgery was performed ("he must not have had a facelift because the plastic surgeon would have surely fixed his baggy eyes").

Fat Grafting in the Male Facelift Patient

A facelift procedure only addresses tissue ptosis and redundancy and often produces a lifted, but telltale hollow, unhealthy, frail, and underrejuvenated "geezer" appearance in men. Fat grafting allows loss of facial fat to be treated simultaneously with the facelift, and these sorts of appearances to be avoided. All things being otherwise equal, simultaneous facelift and fat grafting produces a better result than either technique performed alone, and when a facelift is performed in conjunction with fat grafting loss of facial contour and facial atrophy are corrected, and optimal overall improvement is obtained (**Figs. 44–48**).

Areas in need of treatment vary from patient, but any area that is treated with nonautologous injectable fillers is potentially treatable with fat grafting including, but not limited to, the forehead, temples, radix, upper orbit (upper eyelid), lower orbit (lower eyelid), cheeks, midface, buccal

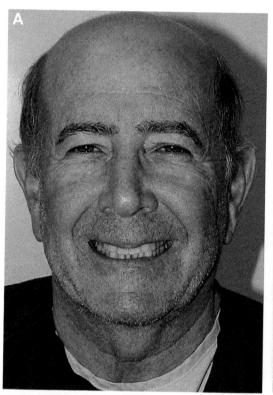
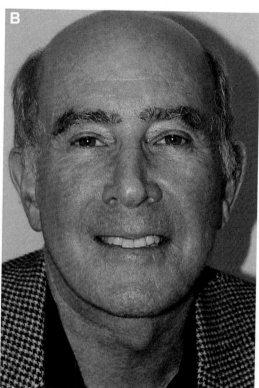

Fig. 45. Patient example 3 (front smiling view). (*A*) Before surgery view of patient, age 68. Note suboptimal upper dental show and tired and disinterested appearance despite broad smile. (*B*) Same patient, 1 year and 9 months after facelift, neck lift, small incision forehead lift, upper and lower eye lifts, partial facial fat grafting, and ear lobe reduction. Note alert and composed appearance and fit, masculine-appearing jawline. A more natural smile with improved dental show is also seen. All surgical procedures performed by Timothy Marten, MD, FACS. (*Courtesy of* Timothy Marten, MD, FACS, San Francisco, CA.)

recess, lips/perioral, nasolabial crease, geniomandibular groove, chin, and jawline areas.

The young attractive, athletic, and masculine face is characterized by not only a full upper and lower orbit, but by a rectangular shape and a strong mandibular contour. Replenishing lost volume along the mandible, although initially counterintuitive, restores a more youthful male facial shape and a more bold and decisive appearance. In addition, a more masculine and eye appealing transition from the face to the neck is obtained (see **Fig. 34**).

It is commonly believed by men that fat grafting their lips feminizes the mouth, but the young, attractive, healthy male mouth is full and replenishing lost perioral volume is an important part of creating a harmonious and natural-appearing rejuvenation of the male face. The key in most cases is filling of the lower lip and photographs of the patient when he was younger are often helpful in explaining the need for lip and orbital fat grafting because these almost uniformly

show a full appearance of those areas. Fat grafting the lips (predominantly the lower lip) combined with upper lip lift is an excellent approach for rejuvenation of the male mouth because it is much less often wrinkled than the mouths of women seeking facelift.

PREOPERATIVE PREPARATIONS IN THE MALE PATIENT

It is important that adequate operating room time be allotted for contemporary facelift procedures in men, because they are deceptively time consuming when compared with lifts performed in women. Most men also present more difficultly in terms of bleeding and hemostasis, and the surgeon typically needs to spend extra time accommodating issues related to beard shift. A SMAS facelift, when performed in conjunction with neck lift, eyelid surgery, fat grafting, and other procedures in a male patient, often encompasses 6 to 8 hours or more, even when performed by a

A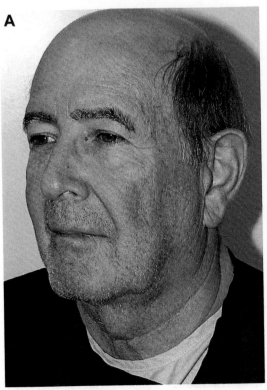

B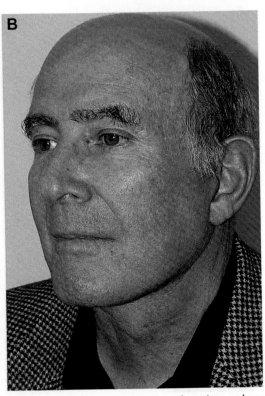

Fig. 46. Patient example 3 (oblique view). (*A*) Before surgery view of patient age 68. Note drooping eyebrow, hooded upper eyelid, sagging cheek, and loss of youthful facial contour. There is little if any transition from the lower cheek to the neck, and a poor jawline is present. (*B*) Same patient, 1 year and 9 months after facelift, neck lift, closed forehead lift, upper and lower eye lifts, partial facial fat grafting, and ear lobe reduction. Note improved eyebrow position and configuration, restoration of cheek fullness, diminished cheek (nasolabial) fold, smooth masculine jawline, and improved neck contour. The patient has a rested, fit, decisive, virile, and masculine appearance. An improved transition from the lower cheek to the neck is evident. All surgical procedures performed by Timothy Marten, MD, FACS. (*Courtesy of* Timothy Marten, MD, FACS, San Francisco, CA.)

"fast" surgeon working with a well-organized and experienced operating room team.

Anesthesia in the Male Facelift Patient

Most of our facelifts are now performed under deep intravenous sedation administered by an anesthesiologist using a laryngeal mask airway. A laryngeal mask allows the patient to be heavily sedated without compromise of their airway, but the patient need not receive muscle relaxants and is allowed to breath spontaneously. In most cases the cuff need not be inflated and is used simply as an oral airway. A laryngeal mask is also less likely to become dislodged during the procedure than an endotracheal tube, and it is less likely to trigger coughing and bucking when the patient's head is turned or when he emerges from the anesthetic. Despite some assertions to the contrary, a laryngeal mask is well suited to long cases, and we have used laryngeal mask airways for 6- to 8-

hour-long procedures for many years without any significant related problems.

Hypertension is common in many men seeking facelifts and male patients are more prone to associated bleeding-related complications, including hematoma, than female patients. As such hypertension must be carefully managed in the perioperative period in male patients. An important part of perioperative management of hypertension is the formulation a proactive plan for preoperative, preemptive treatment and prevention, and most male facelift patients receive a β- blocker (atenolol, 12.5–25 mg orally) and clonidine (0.1–0.3 mg orally) preoperatively. Perioperative blood pressure is then closely monitored and aggressively treated intraoperatively if it becomes elevated (labetalol, 5–10 mg intravenous every 10 minutes as needed), with the goal of operating on a normotensive patient (mean arterial pressure within 10%–15% of preoperative value). Using hypotensive anesthesia, as advocated by some surgeons,

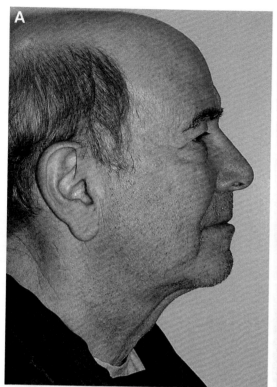 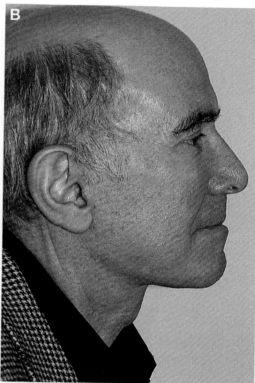

Fig. 47. Patient example 3 (side view). (*A*) Before surgery view of patient age 68. Note lower eyelid puffiness, sagging cheek, poor jawline, heavy jowl, and neck laxity. A protruding salivary gland can also be seen in the neck area. (*B*) Same patient, 1 year and 9 months after facelift, neck lift, closed forehead lift, upper and lower eye lifts, partial facial fat grafting, and ear lobe reduction. An improved transition from the lower eyelid to the upper cheek is seen; the cheek position has been improved; and a fit, masculine-appearing jawline and neckline is evident. The protruding portion of the salivary gland has also been removed. The face has a natural appearance and all scars are well concealed. Note also that the earlobe has been subtly reduced adding to an overall more youthful appearance. All surgical procedures performed by Timothy Marten, MD, FACS. *Courtesy of* Timothy Marten, MD, FACS, San Francisco, CA

carries an increased risk of postoperative bleeding and related complications.

Drain Placement

Drains are routinely used and experience has shown that they reduce postoperative ecchymosis and induration, and allow patients to return to their work and social lives sooner. Two or three 10F catheter round end-perforated Jackson-Pratt style closed-circuit suction drains are typically placed in male patients if neck lift is concomitantly performed. Two drains are typically placed subcutaneously across the anterior-inferior neck on the right and left sides. A third drain is then placed in a similar fashion but pulled into the subplatysmal space. No drains are placed cheeks or face.

Preauricular Beard Follicle Epilation

Before closure of the preauricular portion of the facelift incision an opportunity exists to reduce the beard follicles present on the part of the flap advanced onto the tragus in older men with larger flap shifts. Small skin hooks are used to invert the preauricular skin flap over the surgeon's fingertip. If the patient has 2 to 3 days of beard growth and has not shaved the day of surgery this pushes the beard follicles up out of the subcutaneous fat on the undersurface of the flap. Using loupe magnification, individual follicles are then directly excised with a small serrated scissors (Kaye blepharoplasty scissors) and/or directly epilated using a needle-tipped (Colorado) cautery set on low cautery current. Beard follicles can similarly be removed from a small cuff of skin in the prehelical and perilobular parts of the check skin flap (see **Fig. 35**). Care must be taken to apply the cautery precisely and only to the individual follicles themselves. If current is applied carelessly or at too high a level, or otherwise allowed to flow to the skin, vascular compromise and slough can occur.

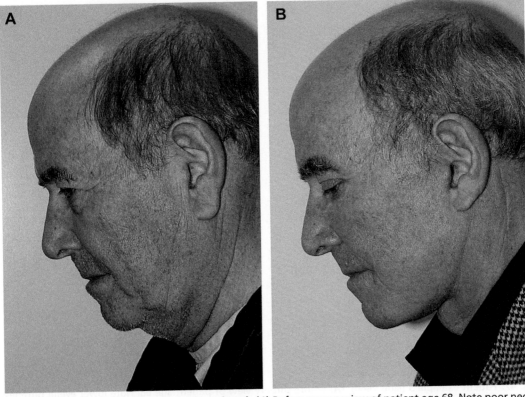

Fig. 48. Patient example 3 (side view, looking down). (*A*) Before surgery view of patient age 68. Note poor neckline when looking down. (*B*) Same patient, 1 year and 9 months after facelift, neck lift, closed forehead lift, upper and lower eye lifts, minor partial facial fat transfer, and ear lobe reduction. Note improved neck contour in the flexed position. The face has a natural appearance and all scars are well concealed. All surgical procedures performed by Timothy Marten, MD, FACS. (*Courtesy of* Timothy Marten, MD, FACS, San Francisco, CA.)

ANCILLARY AND PROCEDURES AND ALTERNATIVE STRATEGIES IN THE MALE PATIENT

Ear Lobe Reduction

Many men presenting for facelift surgery are seen to have overly large earlobes that lend them a telltale old and aged, "grandfatherly" appearance, and reducing them can significantly lighten male facial appearance and improve overall outcomes (**Fig. 36** see also **Figs. 44–48**).

Upper Lip Lift

Many men presenting for facelift surgery are often older than women undergoing the procedure and have a long upper lip (increased vertical distance from the base of the nose to the vermillion-cutaneous junction) and compromised upper dental show when smiling. As such they are excellent candidates for upper lip lift procedures. The beard-skin interface at the base of the nose also provides an excellent location to place and hide the scar in most men.

Nasolabial Fold Excision

Many mature men are seen to have heavy facial skin and deep nasolabial folds with sharp nasolabial creases that are a concern to them, which are minimally improved when even an aggressive facelift is performed, and these patients are candidates for nasolabial fold excision.

Nasolabial fold excision exploits the sharp creases and coarse skin present on many men's faces, and a carefully closed wound results in a scar that is not more conspicuous, or even less conspicuous, that the existing nasolabial crease. Nasolabial fold excision is an excellent procedure for men who have had a previous or recent facelift but have insufficient improvement in their nasolabial fold, men who have modest overall facial laxity but largely isolated nasolabial folds, men with bald or shaved heads that want to avoid a full facelift procedure, and men who are ambivalent about having a preauricular scar.

SUMMARY

Treatment strategies in men are different than those in women and it is not appropriate to arbitrarily apply concepts and techniques that evolved largely for treating the female face to that of a man. The male face is arguably more nuanced than that of a female whom society has come to accept as having a more contrived and made-up appearance, and certain aspects of male facial aging are often regarded as signs of experience, wisdom, and power that many men wish not to lose. In these and other ways men often have different goals than women do when seeking rejuvenation of their faces, with the man arguably more concerned about a natural appearance free of signs that a surgical procedure has been performed. Surgical techniques must be modified accordingly.

CLINICS CARE POINTS

- Male attractiveness is correlated with a more bottom heavy rectangular facial shape, a heavier and bolder jawline, a strong athletic neckline, a lower and more horizontal eyebrow, and a flatter cheek profile.

- Men primarily seek and desire a bold, athletic neckline and jawline, and more subtle and less dramatic changes on other areas of the face.

- A surgeon who can deliver a good result in the neckline and jawline, provide well-concealed scars, and exercise restraint when operating on the forehead, eyes, and mouth, is likely to be successful when treating male patients.

- Many, if not most, of the changes associated with loss of facial contour in men represent primarily deep layer problems that are inadequately corrected if traditional skin-only face and neck lift techniques are used.

- Properly performed, the addition of fat to areas of the male face that have atrophied because of age or disease can produce a significant and sustained improvement in appearance unobtainable by other means.

- In treating the man with the shaved head one can exploit that a key and quintessential feature of an attractive, athletic-appearing man is a good neckline.

- Often men want the improvement afforded by the facelift but cannot get past the name of the procedure. In such cases an accord can usually be struck by simply calling the procedure an extended neck lift and modifying the facelift incision plan slightly accordingly.

DISCLOSURE

The authors have nothing to disclose. The concepts, methods, and technique described and contained in this chapter are the opinions of the authors and are not intended to be construed as, or used to define, a standard of care.

ACKNOWLEDGMENTS

All photographs, illustrations, descriptions and text contained in this article are courtesy of the Timothy Marten, MD, FACS and are used with permission.

REFERENCES

1. Marten, TJ, Elyassnia DR, "Male facelift" In Plastic surgery (4th ed) Neligan, ed 2018
2. Marten TJ, Elyassnia DR. Facial fat grafting : why, where, how, and how much. Aesthet Plast Surg 2018;42:5.
3. Marten TJ, Elyassnia DR. The role of fat grafting in facial rejuvenation. Clin Plast Surg 2015;42:219.
4. Marten, TJ, "Simultaneous facelift and fat grafting". In Fat grafting. Coleman, S, ed. 2017.
5. Marten TJ, Elyassnia DR. Neck lift: defining anatomic problems and choosing appropriate treatment strategies. Clin Plast Surg 2018;45(4):455–84.
6. Marten, TJ, Elyassnia DR, "Secondary necklift". In Aesthetic plastic surgery Foad. Nahai, MD ed 3rd ed 2019.
7. Marten TJ, Elyassnia DR. Neck lift. In: Plastic and Reconstructive surgery. Wiley; 2021.
8. Marten TJ, Elyassnia DR. Management of the platysma in neck lift. Clin Plast Surg 2018;45(4):555–70.
9. Marten TJ, Elyassnia DR, "Lamellar high SMAS face and mid-lift: improved design of the SMAS facelift for better results in the mid-face and infra-orbital region". In Aesthetic plastic surgery Foad. Nahai, MD ed 3nrd ed 2019.
10. Marten TJ. Lamellar high SMAS facelift: simultaneous lifting of the mid-face, cheek and jowl In Paul, M. Clin Plast Surg 2008.
11. Marten, TJ, Elyassnia DR, "Secondary facelift". In Plastic surgery (4th ed) Neligan, ed 2018.
12. Marten TJ. Closed, non-endoscopic, small incision forehead lift. Clin Plast Surg 2008.

13. Connell BF, Marten TJ. "Foreheadplasty for men -recognizing and treating aging in the upper face". Clin Plast Surg 1991.

14. Marten TJ, Elyassnia DR. Forehead lift. In: Plastic and Reconstructive surgery. Wiley; 2021.

15. Marten TJ. In: David Knize MD, editor. Forehead aesthetics and pre-operative Assessment of the foreheadplasty patient" the forehead and temporal fossa: anatomy and technique. Lippincott Williams and Wilkins; 2001.

16. Marten TJ, Elyassnia DR. Short scar neck lift: neck lift using a submental incision only. Clin Plast Surgery 2018.

17. Connell BF, Marten TJ. Facelift for the active man" Instructional Courses in plastic surgery. C.V. Mosby Co.; 1991.

18. Marten TJ. In: David Knize MD, editor. Open foreheadplasty" the forehead and temporal fossa: anatomy and technique. Lippincott Williams and Wilkins; 2001.

Neck Contouring and Rejuvenation in Male Patients Through Dual-Plane Reduction Neck Lift

Francisco G. Bravo, MD, PhD

KEYWORDS

- Neck lift • Face lift • Facial rejuvenation • Cervicofacial rejuvenation • Jawline definition
- Male plastic surgery • Male aesthetics • Submentoplasty

KEY POINTS

- Surgeons seeking successful outcomes in male facial rejuvenation must be able to achieve balanced and natural results in the neck and submental region.
- A thorough understanding of male jawline and neck surface aesthetics and its relevance to perceived age, attractiveness, and body mass index is necessary to plan the best treatment option for cervical enhancement.
- Neck and submental surgical procedures provide better and longer-lasting results when the deep structures of the neck are contoured independently from the redraping maneuvers performed on the superficial layers.
- A dual-plane approach to the neck divides it into a submandibular and a cervical segment, which is managed differently, allowing for more defined and natural outcomes with lower revision rates.
- Indications for neck lift surgery as well as complications arising from it, should be fully understood by specialists providing facial rejuvenation procedures.

INTRODUCTION

With the latest advances and rapid growth in minimally invasive procedures for facial rejuvenation, male patients are showing an increased interest in such techniques.[1] Due to the success of these treatments, patients will often visit the plastic surgeon at a later age when the neck is often the major concern.[2] Although much effort has been devoted to improving the neck and jawline nonsurgically[3] and despite the fact that in general, male patients are often hesitant to undergoing surgical cosmetic procedures for fear of looking unnatural or overdone, surgery is often the best option to obtain significant and long-lasting results in the neck and submental region. Specialists seeking successful outcomes in facial rejuvenation should recognize the importance of the neck to provide their patients with balanced and natural results and avoid an overdone face-underdone neck deformity.[4]

Many patients who are candidates for facelift surgery worry more about the physical changes in the neck than about those in the face and specialists performing facial rejuvenation surgery should use all their ingenuity and skill to obtain optimum results in the neck.[5]

In this regard, the neck is not only an important element to achieve harmony when undertaking any facial rejuvenation procedure but it is also on itself, an important component of both facial aesthetics and youthfulness, and also plays an important role in the perceived body mass appearance of an individual.

The author has no commercial or financial conflict of interest and have received no funding for the preparation and writing of this article.
Clinica Gomez Bravo, Claudio Coello 76, Madrid 28001, Spain
E-mail address: fgbravo@clinicagomezbravo.com

Clin Plastic Surg 49 (2022) 257–273
https://doi.org/10.1016/j.cps.2021.12.002
0094-1298/22/

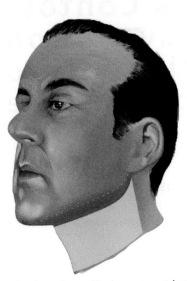

■ Submandibular Cervical (SC) Junction Line

■ Submandibular Segment (Superficial and Deep dissections):
- Subcutaneous Plane
- Subplatysmal Plane

■ Cervical Segment (Deep only dissection):
- Skin-Muscle Attached
- Subplatysmal Plane

Fig. 1. The Submandibular-Cervical Junction Line (*red line*), whereby the submandibular segment (*orange*) and cervical segment (*green*) of the neck meet. In a dual-plane neck lift, each segment is dissected and managed differently. (*Modified from* Bravo FG. Reduction Neck Lift: The Importance of the Deep Structures of the Neck to the Successful Neck Lift. Clin Plast Surg. 2018 Oct;45(4):485-506.)

Careful planning should be undertaken when deciding what techniques to use and which anatomic structures need to be addressed to achieve optimal results in neck contouring, as the management of the deep structures of the neck is often a requirement in modern cervical rejuvenation.[4]

SURFACE AESTHETICS OF THE MALE NECK

A thorough knowledge of the morphologic characteristics of the young and attractive male neck and jawline is essential to understand the surgical maneuvers necessary to mimic those features and design a surgical plan accordingly. Hence, a careful analysis and description of the surface aesthetics of the neck and submandibular region of the male patient, as well as of its underlying anatomy is paramount to achieve good outcomes in neck lift surgery.

A clinically relevant surface landmark when analyzing neck aesthetics is the *submandibular-cervical (SC) junction line,* which lies below the border of the jawline and delineates whereby the submandibular segment of the neck meets the cervical segment (**Fig. 1**). This line serves as the reference point to establish 3 different angles which have significance in cervical aesthetics: (1) the anterior submandibular-cervical angle (ie, the submental-cervical angle), which constitutes the most studied proportion in the neck and that should be around 100° in the attractive young individual, (2) the lateral submandibular-cervical angle, around 120°, and (3) the posterior

submandibular-cervical angle, which should be around 140° (**Fig. 2**).

The submental-cervical angle has been the most studied in the literature[6,7] because it is easily measurable from the profile view. Unfortunately, the lateral and posterior submandibular-cervical angles are less evident, as they can only be analyzed from a postero-cranial or antero-caudal view (**Fig. 3**) and will only be perceived visually by the shadow formed beneath the mandible in the three-quarter and profile views (**Fig. 4**).

There is a general consensus that achieving a well-defined jawline is one of the main objectives of a successful surgical cervicofacial rejuvenation procedure. A well-defined mandible requires that the surface of the lower cheek and jaw, be separated sufficiently from the neck. This separation or depth beneath the border of the mandible allows a shadow to be cast below the full length of the mandible which is a key element in the perception of a well-defined jawline.

The separation of the mandible from the neck is more evident anteriorly as the chin projects more from the neck than any other area of the mandible and the submandibular cervical angle is more acute anteriorly and gradually tapers down along the submandibular-cervical junction line posteriorly. To achieve a successful neck lift, however, depth beneath the mandible should be achieved along its body and angle as well (zones 2 and 3),[4,8] by reducing the submandibular structures at these levels, aiming to provide a shadow underneath the entire length of the jawline, which will greatly define it.

- Mandibular Border

- Submandibular-Cervical Junction Line

- Submental-Cervical Angle (100°)

- Lateral Submandibular-Cervical Angle (120°)

- Posterior Submandibular-Cervical Angle (140°)

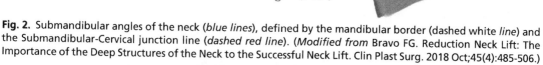

Fig. 2. Submandibular angles of the neck (*blue lines*), defined by the mandibular border (dashed white *line*) and the Submandibular-Cervical junction line (*dashed red line*). (*Modified from* Bravo FG. Reduction Neck Lift: The Importance of the Deep Structures of the Neck to the Successful Neck Lift. Clin Plast Surg. 2018 Oct;45(4):485-506.)

This shadow is seen as an extension of the submental line into the neck when viewed in profile view, forming an *extended submental line,* which is an important feature of the young and attractive neck (**Fig. 5**). Achieving an extended submental line should be an objective when performing neck lift surgery, to obtain a *single crease neck* when the patient looks down, as opposed to a *double crease neck,* which often occurs as a surgical stigma of face and neck lift surgery when the deep submandibular structures are not adequately managed (**Fig. 6**).

Other important features in male neck surface aesthetics are an evident thyroid cartilage protuberance, at an approximate 140° angle with respect to the anterior neck line and a visible sternocleidomastoid muscle line centrally and cranially near the mandible, defining the musculomandibular triangle (**Fig. 7**).

THE NECKS̓ INFLUENCE ON PERCEPTION

Modifying the shape of a specific anatomic structure may have a considerable influence on the way individuals are perceived by others. A thorough understanding of this phenomenon is essential to the plastic surgeon to prioritize which areas need to be addressed first, according to the patients̓ concerns and expectations.

In the case of the neck, its surgical modification may have a significant impact on the way male patients are perceived by others with respect to 3 distinct areas: (1) their apparent age, (2) their attractiveness, and (3) their body mass index or overall physical fitness and body type.

Impact of the Neck on Male Perceived Age: the Impact of Perifacial Versus Centrofacial Morphology on the Overall Perception of Facial Aging

The neck has a profound impact on the overall perception others have of our age. To determine whether morphologic changes occurring at the periphery of the face with aging have more or less of an impact on the overall perception of facial aging than those occurring centrally, the following study was performed[9]: 1171 photographs of 100 male public figures collected from Google Images were analyzed. Public domain images in 3-quarter view were selected and 50 subjects were randomly chosen for the study.

Through imaging software, the central part of the face was swapped between the younger and older versions of each subject. The resulting set of digitally altered images consisted of a young perifacial version with an aged centrofacial area and an elderly perifacial version with a young centrofacial area (**Fig. 8**). Subsequently, 32 individuals were recruited to evaluate the modified images. Each volunteer was asked to select the subject that they considered to be the youngest out of each set of modified images. Statistical analysis of the data was performed, which showed that a significant 61.2% ± 2.6% (*P*<.05) of individuals selected subjects with the youngest perifacial morphology and older centrofacial anatomy as the ones with an overall youngest appearance. 15% of the male subjects studied presented with a predominant facial thinning with aging (Type I aging), while in 85% of the subjects, a predominant perifacial expansion was noted (Type II aging). In both instances, the same conclusion may be drawn from the careful analysis of facial images of individuals as they age: the aging process is devastating.

The finding that most individuals perceive subjects with a more juvenile perifacial area as younger, despite a more elderly centrofacial appearance, may have a significant influence on the direction our specialty should take regarding facial rejuvenation. Efforts on improving perifacial areas such as the jawline and neck despite requiring more complex surgical procedures should remain a key element in the management of the aging face. In conclusion, with respect to facial rejuvenation and just as was the case with

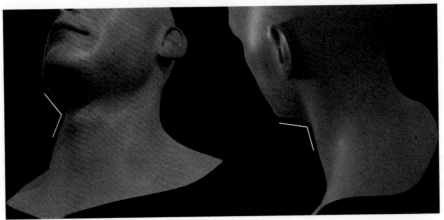

Fig. 3. Antero-caudal (*left*) and postero-cranial (*right*) views, which allow the visualization of the lateral submandibular-cervical angle.

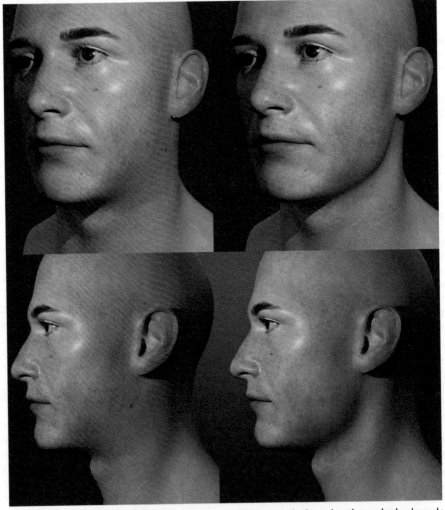

Fig. 4. Appreciation of the lateral and posterior submandibular-cervical angles through shadow depth in the three-quarter (above) and profile (below) views. The 3D models on the right had submandibular volume reduction applied digitally. The same lighting was used for all models.

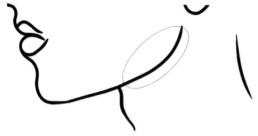

Fig. 5. Extended submental line (*blue oval line*), continuing the submental line into the neck, defining the mandibular border.

the Italian Renaissance, the frame is just as important as the painting itself and the neck lift may be considered as the new face lift.

Impact of the Neck on Male Perceived Attractiveness

Several studies have demonstrated the importance the neck plays when determining the attractiveness of an individual, based on both the submental-cervical angle[6] and on neck ptosis.[10]

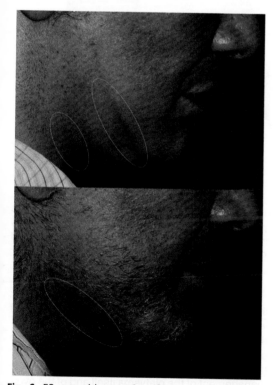

Fig. 6. 52-year-old secondary face and neck lift patient with a double crease neck (*white ovals lines*) before (above) and after (below) a reduction neck lift procedure. Note the achievement of a single crease neck with an extended submental line (*white oval*) after the surgery.

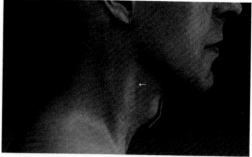

Fig. 7. Surface aesthetics of the male neck with an evident thyroid protuberance at an approximately 140° angle to the anterior cervical line and visible sternocleidomastoid muscle shadow lines centrally and cranially (*white arrow*), blending together with the submandibular shadow to form the musculomandibular triangle.

The neck and jawline also play a very important role in one of the 4 main attributes that influence facial attractiveness: sexual dimorphism (ie, features that accentuate the masculinity of the male individual). The other 3 being averageness, symmetry, and youthfulness.[11,12]

Indeed, a well-defined, cuadrangular, and prominent jawline, together with a noticeable thyroid cartilage protuberance (ie, Adam's apple) are key features of the masculine attractive individual, as evidenced by the fact that they are essential areas targeted in facial gender reassignment surgery.[13,14]

Impact of the Neck on Male Perceived Fitness

Then neck has a significant influence on the apparent body mass index of an individual and their overall fitness and body type. In fact, most patients that have undergone a neck lift procedure remark that the most frequent comment they encounter postoperatively by their acquaintances unaware of their surgery is whether they have lost weight.

The correlation between neck volume and perceived body type is evidenced by the fact that neck circumference is used as a screening method for detecting overweight and obese patients[15] and male individuals with a neck circumference equal or greater than 37 cm may require additional evaluation of overweight or obesity status.[16]

Furthermore, a recent study has also shown an increase in the volume of the submandibular glands with both aging and body mass index.[17]

SURGICAL TECHNIQUE - DUAL-PLANE REDUCTION NECK LIFT

Despite the obvious inclination to attempt minimally invasive neck lift procedures by recontouring

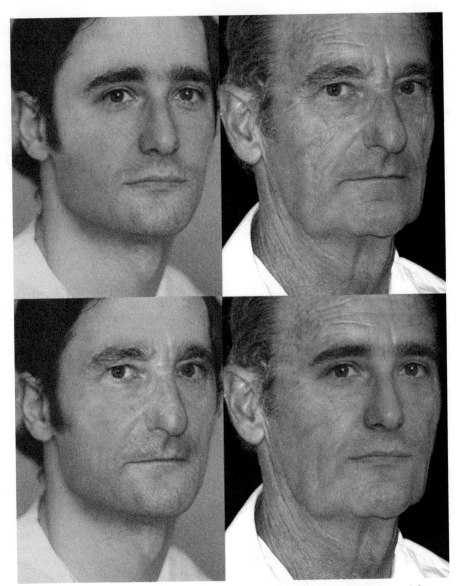

Fig. 8. Young and aged versions (above) of a male individual. The images had their central face swapped between them through digital software (below) and participants were asked to identify which of the 2 photographs depicted an older individual: the one on the lower left (with a young perifacial appearance but aged central face) or the one on the lower right (with a young central face but aged perifacial morphology).

the neck with suspension sutures,[18] it may be more appropriate, to produce long-lasting corrections, to avoid over operating in the superficial planes to improve on deeper problems.[19]

Indeed, although a visible improvement of the submandibular contour may be achieved temporarily by aggressively pulling and tightening the skin and platysma over any protruding subplatysmal structure, a relapse of the submandibular fullness will eventually happen with time, especially in the profile view with the patient looking down (ie, Connel view).

When performing a dual-plane reduction neck lift, 2 distinct goals are pursued and managed independently: (1) volume recontouring or reduction, which is mainly accomplished in the deep structures of the neck beneath the platysma and (2) superficial redraping, which consists of the management of the platysma itself and of the overlying subcutaneous fat and skin under minimal tension.

A dual-plane approach to the neck is used, meaning 2 different dissection planes are carried out. In the area cranial to the SC junction line (ie,

Zone I

- Supraplatysmal fat

- Inter-SCMO fat

- Subplatysmal fat

- Anterior belly of the Digastric Muscles

- Hyoid Release

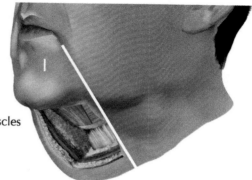

Fig. 9. Submandibular Zone I, below the submental region. The anatomic structures that may be addressed are the supraplatysmal fat, the intersternocleidomastoid origin fat, the subplatysmal fat, the anterior belly of the digastric muscles, and the hyoid. (*Modified from* Bravo FG. Reduction Neck Lift: The Importance of the Deep Structures of the Neck to the Successful Neck Lift. Clin Plast Surg. 2018 Oct;45(4):485-506.)

submandibular segment), a plane is developed both superficial and deep to the platysma, while in the area caudal to this line (ie, cervical segment), dissection is carried out only deep to the platysma, leaving the muscle attached to its overlying skin (see **Fig. 1**).

Deep Work – Volume Contouring and Reduction

Some individuals without excessive submandibular volume may benefit from a tightening face-lift procedure, through the management of the platysma-skin superficial layer alone. However, most male patients with any degree of perifacial expansion or submandibular fullness will have better outcomes with contouring of the deeper structures of the neck through a reduction neck lift.

It is useful to divide the submandibular region toin 3 distinct zones, according to the anatomic structures that need to be addressed to approach them systematically.[4,8]

Zone I

This is the zone underneath the parasymphyseal lines or anterior mental region of the mandible (**Fig. 9**).

A substantial reduction of subplatysmal fat is frequently necessary to obtain results in male neck lift surgery. Not only does this fat account for a considerable amount of the overall soft-tissue volume of the neck[20,21] but also its management through liposuction alone is often not successful, due to its deep location in the neck and its more fibrous consistency.

Resection is best carried out through direct excision by means of an anterior open approach using electrocautery.

Reduction of the anterior belly of the digastric (ABD) muscles may be required to achieve a flat surface under the chin in selected patients presenting with submental fullness. Excessive bulkiness of the ABD muscles, may be assessed both pre- and intraoperatively by tilting the patients head down or bringing the mandible down toward the neck. If muscular bulging occurs, tangential resection with electrocautery through an anterior approach should be considered.

ABD muscle reduction may also be required if both the subplatysmal fat and submandibular gland have also been reduced. Partial resection of these 2 latter structures may make more evident the presence of the ABD muscles in the neck postoperatively; therefore, making it necessary to reduce these muscles as well.

Zone II

This region represents the area below the body of the mandible, between the parasymphysis and angle and its management is key to improve jawline definition (**Fig. 10**).

Most of the volume responsible for submandibular fullness at this level is due to a deep subplatysmal cervical structure, the submandibular gland, which is often enlarged[22,23] and caudally displaced.[24]

Patients with submental fullness will often present with enlarged submandibular glands (SMGs) and partial surgical reduction of the segment of the gland laying below the level of the mandible may significantly improve jawline definition.

Providing depth under the mandible at this level will improve the lateral submandibular-cervical angle allowing a shadow to appear under the lateral jawline and resulting in a more visible anterior edge of the sternocleidomastoid muscle,

Zone II

- Jowl

- Submandibular gland

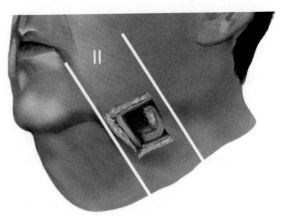

Fig. 10. Submandibular Zone II, below the body of the mandible. The anatomic structures usually managed are the submandibular jowl and the submandibular gland. (*Modified from* Bravo FG. Reduction Neck Lift: The Importance of the Deep Structures of the Neck to the Successful Neck Lift. Clin Plast Surg. 2018 Oct;45(4):485-506.)

which provides a pleasing musculomandibular triangle.

Surgical reduction of the SMGs is better achieved through an anterior submandibular incision posterior to the submental crease,[25–27] although partial reductions may also be performed through a lateral face-lift approach.[28,29]

Zone III

This is the area below and behind the angle of the mandible and it plays an important role in delineating the posterior edge of the jawline, forming the posterior submandibular-cervical angle, and creating a retromandibular hollow or groove (**Fig. 11**).

Superficial fat may be scarce in this area and oftentimes, most of the volume in this zone is due to a prominent tail of parotid gland, which is located deep to the SMAS/platysma plane.[30]

To achieve adequate posterior jawline definition in patients with excessive fullness at this level, partial reduction of the tail of the parotid gland (TPG) may be warranted.[4,26]

Careful SMAS/platysma flap elevation is necessary to expose the parotid gland and to adequately cover the resected area to avoid Freýs Syndrome postoperatively.

Superficial Work - Skin, Subcutaneous Fat, and Platysma Redraping

Once an adequate submandibular contour is achieved through the reduction of the deep structures of the neck, attention is paid to the superficial layers, with the goal of achieving a natural, tension-free redraping of the overlying platysma, subcutaneous fat, and skin.

The work performed superficially is key to achieving a well-padded and even subcutaneous layer in the neck, as well as to preventing platysma

Zone III

- Preplatysmal fat

- Tail of the Parotid Gland

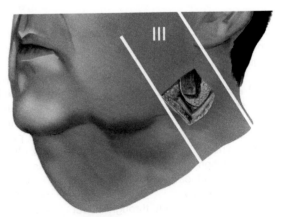

Fig. 11. Submandibular Zone III, below the angle of the mandible. The anatomic structures that may be addressed are the preplatysmal fat and the tail of the parotid gland.

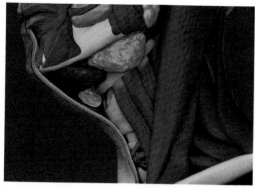

Fig. 12. A patch of subplatysmal fat is shown being left attached to the undersurface of the platysma at the level of the hyoid.

band recurrence and addressing skin laxity or wrinkling in older male patients.

3D Z-Platysmaplasty

The SC junction line is the landmark used to manage the platysma dissection. It must be noted that this line must be marked on the skin below the level of the hyoid preoperatively, as it will end up higher on the neck after the procedure. A lateral traction maneuver performed on the skin of the neck while asking the patient to flex his neck will help identify the patients' SC junction line which divides the neck into a submandibular and a cervical segment.

Along the submandibular segment, the platysma is dissected completely from the skin superficial to it as well as from the deeper subplatysmal structures. Care is taken to preserve a patch of subplatysmal fat attached to the undersurface of the muscle at the level of the hyoid, which will aid in preventing platysma band recurrence (**Fig. 12**). The cervical segment (caudal to the SC junction line) is dissected only deep to the

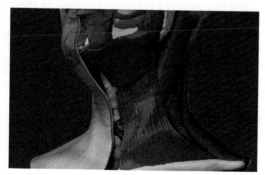

Fig. 13. Full-length, full-thickness horizontal transection of the platysma is shown, which divides the platysma into cranial and caudal portions.

platysma, leaving the skin and subcutaneous fat attached to the muscle superficially.

The platysma is transected horizontally, full-length and full-thickness along the preoperative SC junction line (below the hyoid), dividing the platysma into a cranial and a caudal segment (**Fig. 13**). The deep cervical fascia is also transected at this level, taking care not to injure the anterior cervical veins and its communicating branches to the external jugular vein, which run immediately beneath it. The purpose of this is twofold: (1) it completely separates the cranial and caudal platysma segments, preventing the transmission of forces with muscle contraction through the deep cervical fascia, which may cause dynamic band recurrence[31] and (2) it allows for the denervation of the caudal platysma segment by injury to the cervical branch of the facial nerve which runs deep to the platysma laterally.[32] This caudal denervation of the platysma not only decreases the incidence of platysma band recurrence but also enhances the overlying skin quality considerably through a surgical "botulinum toxin effect" (**Fig. 14**).

To avoid platysma band recurrence a Z-plasty approach is planned, as it generally constitutes the best option to treat scar bands and skin webbing in plastic surgery. Other authors have proposed the use of Z-plasties for midline platysma plication.[33,34] The method proposed here is different and is based on a 3D Z-plasty concept, consisting in separating the cranial and caudal segment of each medial platysma band as far away from each other as possible through opposing vectors, following the x, y, and z axis of 3D space (**Fig. 15**).

Midline plication of the cranial platysma segments is performed with interrupted resorbable sutures, anchoring the medial edges of the platysma both to the anterior belly of the digastrics[35] and to the hyoid bone.[36,37] Excess platysma, when present, may be trimmed vertically before performing the plication or horizontally if bowstringing of the platysma is observed.

The caudal inter-platysma fat, which is attached to the skin and medial edges of the caudal platysma segments, is suspended vertically and anchored to the hyoid to provide adequate soft tissue padding of the thyroid cartilage and prevent medial window shading of the platysma.

Laterally, the cranial platysma segment is tightened through an inter-locking cable suture anchored to the mastoid. This suture may further define and provide depth to Zone 3, once both the superficial fat and the most posterior-caudal portion of the submandibular gland have been reduced and as long as the tail of the parotid gland

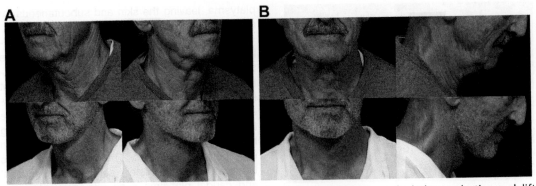

Fig. 14. (*A*, *B*) 72-year-old-patient before (above) and after (below) undergoing a dual-plane reduction neck lift. Notice the improvement in skin wrinkling and quality after the surgical denervation of the caudal portion of the platysma and the correction of the thick platysma bands through 3D Z-platysmaplasty.

is not overly hypertrophic. The caudal platysma segment, with its overlying attached skin, is also anchored to the mastoid region through 2 interlocking cable sutures, shifting both the muscle and skin together as a unit, in a similar fashion as other authors have described previously,[28,29] but applying this composite flap concept only to the caudal platysma (ie, below the SC junction line).

Subcutaneous Fat Management

Reduction of superficial subcutaneous fat should be carried out judiciously and devised as a means of fine-tuning the desired outcome. Maintaining sufficiently thick padding of subcutaneous fat attached to the undersurface of the elevated skin flap in the neck is key to achieve a soft and natural result, avoiding a skeletonized look and reducing the risk of skin adherences or irregularities, which may be difficult to correct secondarily.

Zone 1 is usually the area with the most amount of superficial fat accumulation. Excision is carried

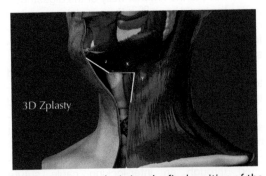

Fig. 15. Illustration depicting the final position of the medial border of the platysma responsible for vertical band formation after 3D Z-platysmaplasty. Notice the separation of the cranial and caudal edges of the platysma in opposing directions, forming a Z configuration along the 3 planes of 3D space: x, y, and z.

out through en-bloc resection using electrocautery, taking care not to injure the underlying platysma muscle.

Although most of the volume in Zone 2 is often due to a prominent submandibular gland, a submandibular jowl may also be present at this level, and must be managed either by direct excision (jowlectomy), microliposuction with 1 cc syringes, and blunt fine-tip cannulas or resuspension into the face.

Finally, in Zone 3, much of the volume present is often due to a large tail of the parotid gland, oftentimes an adequate improvement may be achieved without the need to address the gland by reducing the subcutaneous fat overlying the platysma, which is firmly attached to it in this zone. As mentioned previously, care should be taken not to injure the underlying platysma when resecting the fat in this area with electrocautery or scissors.

Skin Redraping

The final step performed in the superficial layer is the redraping of the skin, which is achieved by applying a hemostatic net at the end of the procedure and leaving it in place for at least 48 hours postoperatively.[38] The use of this technique has 4 main purposes: (1) skin redistribution along the submandibular segment of the neck, extending into the jawline and mastoid area, (2) hematoma and seroma prevention, avoiding the need for drains, dressings or compression garments, (3) improvement of the vascular supply to the skin flap, avoiding excessive tension at the wound edges by redistributing tension along the flap, (4) serve as an added anchoring mechanism to the cable sutures used, by implementing a belt-suspender concept, and (5) reduce the postoperative recovery time and downtime, by diminishing bruising and swelling.

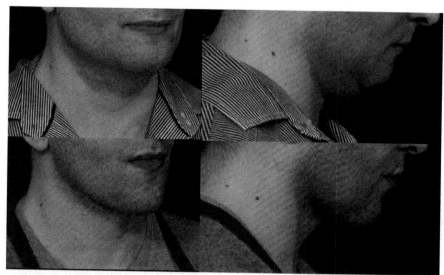

Fig. 16. 29-year-old patient before (above) and after (below) a dual-plane reduction neck lift procedure through and anterior approach only (short-scar neck lift) after unsuccessful laser liposuction was performed elsewhere, which left him with an underdone neck deformity. The patient also had silicone implants placed previously at the angle of the mandible, which were removed transorally at the time of the neck procedure.

COMPLICATIONS
Sialocele

The subcutaneous accumulation of saliva due to the partial resection of the SMGs may occur in approximately 2% of patients undergoing this technique.[39] Management is performed by serial percutaneous aspiration in the office. Botulinum toxin may be applied directly on the gland prophylactically in the operating room or postoperatively after draining the collection once it has occurred.

A temporary hemostatic net may also be applied under local anesthesia in the office to occlude dead space while the sialocele resolves. Recommending a salivary resting diet during the early postoperative period may greatly reduce the incidence of this complication. Such a diet includes restriction in the mastication of solid foods and avoidance of foods that may be excessively salty, sour, spicy, or sweet.[40]

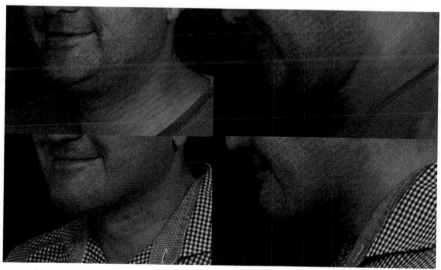

Fig. 17. 38-year-old patient before (above) and after (below) a dual-plane reduction neck lift procedure through and anterior approach (short-scar neck lift). Small perilobular incisions were also used to partially reduce prominent tails of both parotid glands.

Xerostomia

Partial SMG reduction during neck lift surgery does not result in dry mouth syndrome.[39] Studies that have presented an association of SMG resection with this complication belong to the oncologic literature, whereby complete SMG excision is performed in the setting of head and neck cancer. Most of these patients also receive oral radiotherapy, which accounts for the high incidence of xerostomia they refer.[41]

Lower Lip Depressor Weakness

Although temporary weakness of the depressors of the corner of the mouth may occur due to injury to the marginal mandibular branch of the facial nerve during SMG reduction in up to 9% of patients, these numbers are related to transcutaneous complete resections performed directly over the gland in the setting of pathologic or tumoral disorders.[42] Partial gland reductions performed at the moment of face-lift surgery, present with transient depressor weakness rates of up to 4%, which are similar to those occurring in face-lift procedures overall without SMG reduction.[39] Such a complication is more likely related to general face-lift maneuvers such as the release of the mandibular osteocutaneous retaining ligament, which is in close anatomic relationship to the terminal branches of the marginal mandibular branch of the facial nerve.[43] Other mechanisms may be related to the participation of the platysma as a lower lip depressor and its possible transient denervation during platysmaplasty maneuvers,[44] although this influence has also been questioned previously.[32]

Hematoma

Although the risk of a postoperative hematoma after neck lift surgery has been greatly reduced due to the application of the hemostatic net during the early postoperative period,[38] partial excision of the SMG should only be attempted if a possible profuse intraoperative or early postoperative bleeding may be adequately managed, due to the close relationship of the facial artery and common facial vein to the gland.

Prolonged Swelling

A long recovery time, occasionally associated with stiffness and a frozen neck deformity, has usually been attributed to the open neck approach through a submental incision when extensive deep work and skin undermining is performed. The use of the hemostatic net[38] combined with the dual-plane concept, whereby skin undermining is limited to the submandibular segment of the neck, provide recovery times similar to those obtained with lateral-only approaches.

Inadequate Aesthetic Outcome

Several inappropriate intraoperative clinical decisions or postoperative problems may hinder the final result and require surgical revisions:

1. Platysma band recurrence may emerge early in the postoperative period. A correct diagnosis is necessary, as different causes may mimic this entity and not be true recurrences of the initial platysma band. Irregular subcutaneous fat accumulation, prominent anterior belly of the digastric muscles, skin adherences to the underlying platysma as well as skin webbing over the SC junction line may all be erroneously considered as recurrent bands. Prevention may be achieved by the implementation of the 3D Z-platysmaplasty concept described previously, including the elevation of the medial edges of the platysma together with a patch of subplatysmal fat to avoid medial skin adherence to the muscle; adequate fixation of the medial platysma edges both to the digastric muscles and to the hyoid bone to avoid cheese wiring of the midline plethysmography; suspension of the caudal inter-platysma fat to the hyoid to ensure the SC junction line is covered by an adequate layer of subcutaneous fat and platysma that will avoid skin webbing; and denervation of the caudal segment of the platysma, through horizontal deep cervical fascia transection and cervical branch of the facial nerve injury, to improve skin quality and wrinkling of the cervical segment of the neck, as well as achieve relaxation of the medial platysma bands. In any case, the threshold for revising a recurrent band should be very low, as oftentimes it may be performed under local anesthesia and thanks to the use of a local submental hemostatic net,[38] the recovery is usually very fast.

2. An underdone neck deformity may be the most prevalent problem after neck enhancement procedures, as evidenced by the significant differences between the desired submental-cervical angle of patients compared with those proposed by specialists providing treatments in this region.[6] Furthermore, many specialists manage the neck through submental liposuction only, not addressing muscle laxity or prominent subplatysmal structures, which are more evident in a flexed neck position, not usually presented in side-by-side pre- and

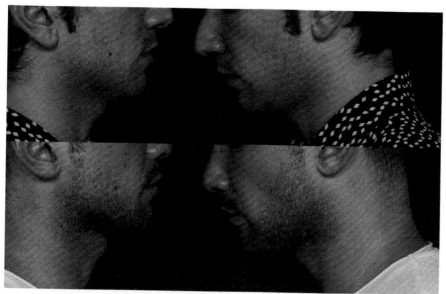

Fig. 18. Young 27-year-old patient before (above) and after (below) a dual-plane reduction neck lift procedure through and anterior approach only (short-scar neck lift). The patient also underwent a closed preservation rhinoplasty with push down of the dorsum and an earlobe reduction.

postoperative images (**Fig. 16**). In other cases, open approaches may have been used through a submental incision, but inadequate management of the deep structures of the neck, together with excessive tension applied to the face, may produce an overdone face-underdone neck deformity yielding a double-crease neck (see **Fig. 6**).

3. Overdone-skeletonized neck deformities may occur after neck lift surgery and may be difficult to repair postoperatively, despite modern fat grafting techniques. Although often attributed to subplatysmal maneuvers such as SMG reduction or shaving of the anterior belly of the digastric muscles, the majority of such cases are actually secondary to excessive

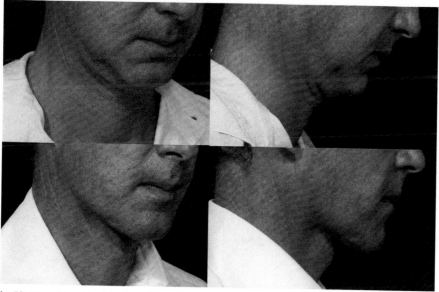

Fig. 19. Thin 53-year-old patient before (above) and after (below) a dual-plane reduction neck lift procedure through and anterior approach only (short-scar neck lift). Reduction of the deep subplatysmal structures was also performed to achieve redraping of the skin and platysma under no tension.

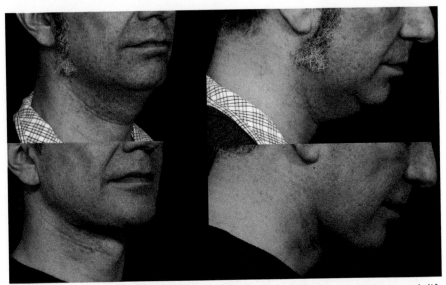

Fig. 20. Thin 41-year-old patient before (above) and after (below) a dual-plane reduction neck lift procedure through and anterior approach only (short-scar neck lift). Reduction of the deeper structures of the neck was necessary to adequately contour the submental region and neck, before tightening the platysma.

resection of subcutaneous fat in the neck or failure to leave sufficient subplatysmal fat over the hyoid and thyroid cartilages to provide for a soft and natural submental-cervical angle.

4. A cobra neck deformity is the result of excessive debulking of the subcutaneous and subplatysmal fat in Zone 1 without adequately addressing the paramedian volume in the neck usually caused by prominent submandibular glands. This produces depression or divot

centrally in the neck and often requires reduction of the submandibular glands and anterior belly of the digastric muscles to correct.

INDICATIONS
Heavy, Thick, Obtuse Neck Patients

Patients with large neck circumferences and abundant submandibular volume are excellent candidates for a dual-plane reduction neck lift procedure. These men often require addressing large

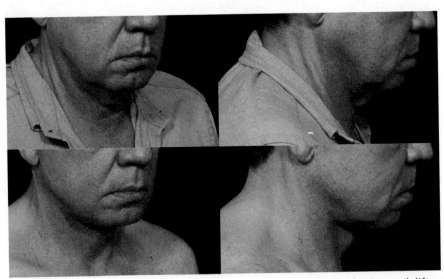

Fig. 21. Thin 59-year-old patient before (above) and after (below) a dual-plane reduction neck lift procedure in which both lateral and anterior approaches were performed. After adequate contouring of the deeper structures, the platysma and skin were redraped under minimal tension extending to the retroauricular area.

subplatysmal structures and often result in high satisfaction rates after the procedure, not only because of their rejuvenated look and enhanced attractiveness thanks to a better-defined jawline and thyroid cartilage protuberance (Adam's apple) but also because of the slimmed-down appearance they portray (**Fig. 17**).

Secondary Facelift or Postsubmental Liposuction Patients

Patients that have previously gone through either a submental liposuction or an open neck lift procedure with unsatisfactory results due to an underdone neck deformity (see **Fig. 16**) or a double-crease neck deformity (see **Fig. 6**) are good candidates for a secondary neck lift procedure addressing the deep structures of the neck and platysma adequately.

Young Patients

Younger patients who might complain of lack of jawline definition or excessive submandibular fullness or that might consult for a possible chin implant placement in the setting of a rhinoplasty procedure may benefit from a short scar isolated neck lift through a submental incision only, using the techniques described previously. These young individuals are usually good candidates as they are often slim and a well-defined neck and jawline is well suited for their complexion (**Fig. 18**).

Older Patients

Despite the general notion that an excessively well-defined jawline and neck may look unnatural in older patients, these individuals, especially if they are fit and active, will greatly benefit from an improved neck appearance, as this is usually the area most affected by aging and despite producing a large impact on perceived age, it usually does not have an effect identifying traits, which usually lie on other anatomic structures such as the eyes or mouth, so the patient will seem younger but not look different (see **Fig. 14**).

Thin Patients with Skin Laxity

Thin patients without excessive submandibular volume may benefit from a dual-plane reduction neck lift procedure through an anterior-only approach (**Figs. 19** and **20**) or by combining anterior and lateral approaches when more skin laxity and poor skin quality is present (**Fig. 21**). Reduction of the deeper structures of the neck and adequate platysma management medially and laterally when necessary ensures a more long-lasting and defined result by minimizing any

tension on the superficial layers from the deep structures with neck movement.

SUMMARY

With the recent rise of nonsurgical and minimally invasive facial procedures, the neck lift has become the cornerstone of facial rejuvenation surgery.[45,46] Plastic surgeons offering surgical solutions in this area are expected to deliver results and these are often best achieved through direct surgical reduction of the deep structures of the neck and adequate management of the superficial layers, including the skin and platysma.

A thorough understanding of the surface aesthetics of the neck and submandibular region, as well as of the relevant anatomic structures susceptible to contouring is essential to providing male patients with successful outcomes in cervicofacial rejuvenation.

The dual-plane reduction neck lift presented may be a useful technique to providing long-lasting, natural results for a variety of male patients seeking enhancement of this important anatomic region.

CLINICS CARE POINTS

- A careful evaluation and analysis of the neck should be carried out in all male patients seeking facial rejuvenation procedures, as improvement in this region has important benefits in male apparent age, attractiveness, and fitness.

- Contouring and reduction of the deep subplatysmal structures of the neck are often necessary to achieve natural and long-lasting results in male surgical facial rejuvenation.

- A dual-plane dissection of the neck together with the use of modern skin redraping techniques broadens the indications for neck lift procedures in male patients and reduces complications while shortening recovery times despite the use of an anterior open submental approach.

REFERENCES

1. Aesthetic plastic surgery national databank statistics 2020. Aesthet Surg J 2021;41:1–16.
2. Stuzin JM. Discussion: a comparison of the full and short-scar face-lift incision techniques in multiple

sets of identical twins. Plast Reconstr Surg 2016; 137:1715–7.

3. Lawrence WT, Plastic Surgery Educational Foundation DATA Committee. Nonsurgical face lift. Plast Reconstr Surg 2006;118:541–5.

4. Bravo FG. Reduction neck lift: the importance of the deep structures of the neck to the successful neck lift. Clin Plast Surg 2018;45:485–506.

5. Guerrero-Santos J, Espaillat L, Morales F. Muscular lift in cervical rhytidoplasty. Plast Reconstr Surg 1974;54:127–30.

6. Naini FB, Cobourne MT, McDonald F, et al. Submental-cervical angle: perceived attractiveness and threshold values of desire for surgery. J Maxillofac Oral Surg 2016;15:469–77.

7. Ellenbogen R, Karlin JV. Visual criteria for success in restoring the youthful neck. Plast Reconstr Surg 1980;66:826–37.

8. O'Daniel TG. Optimizing outcomes in neck lift surgery. Aesthet Surg J 2021;41(8):871–92.

9. Bravo FG. The impact of perifacial vs centrofacial morphology on the overall perception of facial aging. In: The Aesthetic Meeting. Montreal, Canada: American Society for Aesthetic Plastic Surgery (ASAPS); 2015.

10. Forte AJ, Andrew TW, Colasante C, et al. Perception of age, attractiveness, and tiredness after isolated and combined facial subunit aging. Aesthet Plast Surg 2015;39:856–69.

11. Rhodes G. The evolutionary psychology of facial beauty. Annu Rev Psychol 2006;57:199–226.

12. Cunningham MR, Barbee AP, Pike CL. What do women want? Facialmetric assessment of multiple motives in the perception of male facial physical attractiveness. J Pers Soc Psychol 1990;59:61–72.

13. Sykes JM, Dilger AE, Sinclair A. Surgical facial esthetics for gender affirmation. Dermatol Clin 2020; 38:261–8.

14. Capitán L, Gutiérrez Santamaría J, Simon D, et al. Facial gender confirmation surgery: a protocol for diagnosis, surgical planning, and postoperative management. Plast Reconstr Surg 2020;145: 818e–28e.

15. Pei X, Liu L, Imam MU, et al. Neck circumference may be a valuable tool for screening individuals with obesity: findings from a young Chinese population and a meta-analysis. BMC Public Health 2018; 18:529.

16. Ben-Noun L, Sohar E, Laor A. Neck circumference as a simple screening measure for identifying overweight and obese patients. Obes Res 2001;9:470–7.

17. Sawan T, Tower JI, Gordon NA, et al. The submandibular gland and the aging neck: a longitudinal volumetric study. Aesthet Plast Surg 2021;45: 987–91.

18. Giampapa VC, Mesa JM. Neck rejuvenation with suture suspension platysmaplasty technique: a minimally invasive neck lift technique that addresses all patients' anatomic needs. Clin Plast Surg 2014; 41:109–24.

19. Nahai F. Reconsidering neck suspension sutures. Aesthet Surg J 2004;24:365–7.

20. Raveendran SS, Anthony DJ, Ion L. An anatomic basis for volumetric evaluation of the neck. Aesthet Surg J 2012;32:685–91.

21. Larson JD, Tierney WS, Ozturk CN, et al. Defining the fat compartments in the neck: a cadaver study. Aesthet Surg J 2014;34:499–506.

22. Mahne A, El-Haddad G, Alavi A, et al. Assessment of age-related morphological and functional changes of selected structures of the head and neck by computed tomography, magnetic resonance imaging, and positron emission tomography. Semin Nucl Med 2007;37:88–102.

23. Saito N, Sakai O, Bauer CM, et al. Age-related relaxo-volumetric quantitative magnetic resonance imaging of the major salivary glands. J Comput Assist Tomogr 2013;37:272–8.

24. Lee MK, Sepahdari A, Cohen M. Radiologic measurement of submandibular gland ptosis. Facial Plast Surg 2013;29:316–20.

25. Singer DP, Sullivan PK. Submandibular gland I: an anatomic evaluation and surgical approach to submandibular gland resection for facial rejuvenation. Plast Reconstr Surg 2003;112:1150–4 [discussion 1155].

26. Bravo FG. Submandibular and parotid gland reduction in facelift surgery. Plast Reconstr Surg 2013; 132:95–6.

27. Mendelson BC, Tutino R. Submandibular gland reduction in aesthetic surgery of the neck: review of 112 consecutive cases. Plast Reconstr Surg 2015;136:463–71.

28. Gonzalez R. The LOPP-lateral overlapping plication of the platysma: an effective neck lift without submental incision. Clin Plast Surg 2014;41:65–72.

29. Pelle-Ceravolo M, Angelini M, Silvi E. Treatment of anterior neck aging without a submental approach: lateral skin-platysma displacement, a new and proven technique for platysma bands and skin laxity. Plast Reconstr Surg 2017;139:308–21.

30. Feldman J. Neck lift. Stuttgart, Germany: Thieme; 2006.

31. Ellenbogen R, Karlin JV. Regrowth of platysma following platysma cervical lift: etiology and methodology of prevention. Plast Reconstr Surg 1981;67: 616–23.

32. Sinno S, Thorne CH. Cervical branch of facial nerve: an explanation for recurrent platysma bands following necklift and platysmaplasty. Aesthet Surg J 2019;39:1–7.

33. Weisman PA. Simplified technique in submental lipectomy. Plast Reconstr Surg 1971;48:443–6.

34. Guerrerosantos J. Managing platysma bands in the aging neck. Aesthet Surg J 2008;28:211–6.

35. Citarella ER, Condé-Green A, Sinder R. Triple suture for neck contouring: 14 years of experience. Aesthet Surg J 2010;30:311–9.

36. Le Louarn C. Hyo neck lift: preliminary report. Ann Chir Plast Esthet 2016;61:110–6.

37. Yousif NJ, Matloub HS, Sanger JR. Hyoid suspension neck lift. Plast Reconstr Surg 2016;138: 1181–90.

38. Auersvald A, Auersvald LA. Hemostatic net in rhytidoplasty: an efficient and safe method for preventing hematoma in 405 consecutive patients. Aesthet Plast Surg 2014;38:1–9.

39. Benslimane F, Kleidona IA, Cintra HPL, et al. Partial removal of the submaxillary gland for aesthetic indications: a systematic review and critical analysis of the evidence. Aesthet Plast Surg 2020;44:339–48.

40. Marten T. Neck lift: defining anatomical problems and applying logical solutions. Las Vegas, USA: ASAPS Facial and Rhinoplasty Symposium; 2018.

41. Jaguar GC, Lima EN, Kowalski LP, et al. Impact of submandibular gland excision on salivary gland function in head and neck cancer patients. Oral Oncol 2010;46:349–54.

42. Preuss SF, Klussmann JP, Wittekindt C, et al. Submandibular gland excision: 15 years of experience. J Oral Maxillofac Surg 2007;65:953–7.

43. O'Daniel TG. Understanding deep neck anatomy and its clinical relevance. Clin Plast Surg 2018;45: 447–54.

44. Ellenbogen R. Pseudo-paralysis of the mandibular branch of the facial nerve after platysmal face-lift operation. Plast Reconstr Surg 1979;63:364–8.

45. Stuzin JM. Discussion: a comparison of the full and short-scar face-lift incision techniques in multiple sets of identical twins. Plast Reconstr Surg 2016; 137:1715–7.

46. Pezeshk RA, Sieber DA, Rohrich RJ. Neck rejuvenation through the lateral platysma window: a key component of face-lift surgery. Plast Reconstr Surg 2017;139:865–6.

Improving Male Chin and Mandible Eesthetics

David M. Straughan, MD[a],*, Michael J. Yaremchuk, MD[b]

KEYWORDS

• Mandibular implants • Chin implants • Genioplasty • CAD/CAM • Sexual dimorphism

KEY POINTS

- The chin and mandible are distinct in sexual dimorphism.
- Relative to the female, the male mandible has a longer ramus, more acute gonial angle, wider bigonial distance, and a more squared, projecting chin.
- Onlays of alloplastic material on the chin and mandible can augment skeletal contours to simulate the ideal masculine jawline.
- Appropriate evaluation, design, exposure, and surgical technique optimize surgical success.

 Video content accompanies this article at http://www.plasticsurgery.theclinics.com.

INTRODUCTION

The skeleton is a vital determinant of facial attractiveness. The size and shape of the chin and mandible specifically contribute to this as they are fundamental to sexual dimorphism. In general, the male mandible has a longer ramus, more acute gonial angle, increased gonial width, and a more squared and projecting chin when compared with that of the female[1] (**Fig. 1**). Because of this, deficiencies in the chin and mandible can distract from the male esthetic. Therefore, augmentation of these skeletal deficiencies can simulate the ideal masculine jawline and improve overall facial esthetics. Onlay of alloplastic material as well as osteotomy with bone rearrangement are 2 proposed mechanisms to accomplish these goals. This article will focus on the evaluation, preoperative work-up, and surgical techniques to optimize results when undertaking mandibular skeletal augmentation in the male patient.

DISCUSSION
Evaluation

Physical examination

Physical examination is the most important element of preoperative assessment and planning. The first step in the evaluation process is to recognize facial asymmetry. Facial asymmetry is very common, even if it is subclinical.[2] Recognition of these specific asymmetries preoperatively is important to both the surgeon and the patient. They should be identified and discussed during the preoperative consultation so that the patient can anticipate asymmetry in the postoperative result. Preoperatively, these asymmetries belong to the patient. Postoperatively, if not identified before the surgery, they are attributed to the surgeon. Furthermore, as asymmetries become more severe, it is important to recognize that they are more complex than relative skeletal deficiencies or excesses. Rather, they reflect 3-dimensional differences that are most

Funding: There were no external funding sources for this article.
[a] Division of Plastic and Reconstructive Surgery, Massachusetts General Hospital, 55 Fruit Street, WACC 435, Boston, MA 02114, USA; [b] Division of Plastic and Reconstructive Surgery, Massachusetts General Hospital, 170 Commonwealth Avenue, Boston, MA 02116, USA
* Corresponding author.
E-mail address: David.M.Straughan@gmail.com
Twitter: @DrYaremchuk (M.J.Y.)

Clin Plastic Surg 49 (2022) 275–283
https://doi.org/10.1016/j.cps.2021.12.004

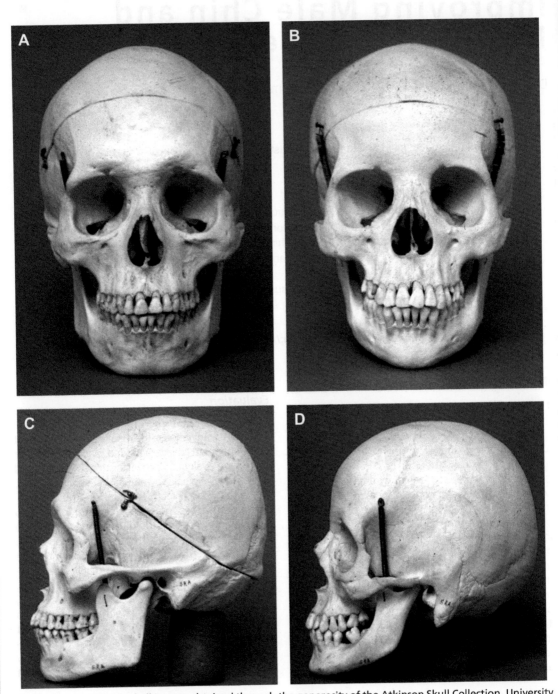

Fig. 1. Female and male skull images obtained through the generosity of the Atkinson Skull Collection, University of the Pacific School of Dentistry, Webster Street, San Francisco, CA, USA. (*A, B*) demonstrate the frontal views of the male and female skulls, respectively. (*C, D*) demonstrate the lateral views of the male and female skulls, respectively. (*From* Yaremchuk MJ. Chapter 2: Evaluation and planning for facial implant surgery. In: Yaremchuk, MJ, ed. Atlas of Facial Implants, 2nd ed. Elsevier; 2020:13-22.)

easily conceptualized as twists of the facial skeleton.

In addition to facial asymmetry, the physical examination should make note of skin quality and prior surgical incisions and scars, as this may alter the surgical procedure. For example, if a prior intraoral incision was placed too close to the sulcus, the surgeon may choose to perform an external approach to the mandible to prevent future healing complications and subsequent implant contamination.

Finally, the examination should focus on the deficiencies of the mandible. Reviewing photographic images with the patient can be helpful when discussing esthetic concerns and goals. When assessing men from the frontal view, the ramus should extend to the level of the oral commissure, and the mandibular angle should project to the level of the lateral orbital rim. From the profile, the mandibular angle should approximate 130°, and the chin should at least project to a point approximately 3° behind a perpendicular line drawn straight down from the glabella.[3,4]

Imaging

Preoperative radiographic imaging is uncommon for pure esthetic surgery. However, it is helpful for facial skeletal surgery. Cephalometric x-rays are most often used for planning chin and mandibular augmentation surgery. These studies define skeletal dimensions and asymmetries as well as the thickness of the chin pad.

Computed tomographic (CT) evaluation provides the ability to view the skeleton in different planes and, through computer manipulation, in 3 dimensions. CT imaging provides digitized information that can be transferred to design software. Computer-aided designed and computer-aided manufactured (CAD/CAM) implants provide an increased level of refinement in both reconstructive and esthetic applications.[5] CAD/CAM can provide implants customized for the specific needs of the patient. The design process can also be conducted virtually.

Cone beam CT scans are available in many dental offices. They have the advantages of less expense and less radiation exposure to the patient.[6] However, because their field is limited and head positioning devices distort the soft tissue envelope, cone beam CT has a limited role in the CAD/CAM implant process.

Facial measurements

Because implant augmentation of the facial skeleton results in measurable changes in facial dimensions and proportions, it is intuitively appropriate to use facial measurements to evaluate the face and to guide surgery. Rather than neoclassical canons, however, facial anthropometrics and the objective data of sexual dimorphism guide the design of male chin and mandible augmentation.

Facial anthropometrics

Anthropometric data aid facial evaluation and surgical planning by describing normal facial measurements and relations. These data provide the average or "normal" dimensions of the face and its component features. Purely esthetic

male chin and mandible surgery most often involves increasing the size and contour of these structures to provide a more masculine appearance. Facial implants must be appropriately sized, shaped, and positioned to be effective. Implants that are too small can result in a less masculinized result, whereas implants that are too large can create unnatural contours that relate poorly to other areas of the face and can ultimately upset facial balance.

Sexual dimorphism

On average, all facial measurements are greater in men than in women. In addition, the relationship between different facial measurements also differs in men and women. These differences are more pronounced in the lower third of the face. For example, the bigonial distance, the lower transverse facial dimension, has the greatest difference between the sexes. In other words, the lower one-third of men's faces tends to be absolutely and relatively wider than that of women.

Esthetic limitations of skeletal osteotomy and rearrangement

Sliding genioplasty and sagittal split osteotomy, which require skills in bone carpentry, can increase the contours of the deficient chin and mandible. However, because no bone is added after osteotomy and rearrangement, the structure remains deficient but in a different way. These deficiencies manifest as gaps at the osteotomy sites resulting in contour irregularities.[5] As a result, the chin often looks "stuck-on" after sliding genioplasty. Because occlusion guides the rearrangement after the sagittal split osteotomy, ramus height and angle width are often asymmetric. For these reasons, alloplastic implants are preferred for esthetic augmentation of the male chin and mandible.

Esthetic limitations of soft tissue augmentation

Soft tissue facial envelope augmentation with autologous fat or filler materials can camouflage underlying minor skeletal irregularities. Whereas augmenting the facial skeleton results in an increase in the projection of the skeleton, augmentation of the soft tissue volume results in an inflation of the soft tissue envelope and blunting of the contours of the skeleton.[7] Fundamentally, these modalities are antipodal in their visual effects. For example, if overly large implants were placed on the skeleton, the appearance would be too defined and ultimately, skeletal. However, excessive fat grafting placed in the soft tissue envelope would result in an increasingly spherical and otherwise amorphous shape.

Esthetic limitation of autogenous bone grafts

Autogenous bone has long been considered the standard material to restore or improve the craniofacial skeleton because it has the potential to be revascularized and assimilate into the facial skeleton. In time, it could be biologically indistinguishable from the adjacent native skeleton. These attributes make it ideal and the only material available to reliably reconstruct segmental load-bearing defects of the facial skeleton. When used as onlay grafts, however, these attributes lead to graft resorption and unreliable, asymmetric augmentation of the facial skeleton.[8]

Implant materials

Silicone rubber, porous polyethylene, and polyetheretherketone (PEEK) are the most commonly used alloplastic implant materials. Each material has advantages and disadvantages. Silicone rubber has a smooth surface and is relatively flexible making implant placement and removal beneath the soft tissue envelope easier. However, its lack of rigidity allows its shape to be distorted by soft tissue deforming forces and makes it feel less like actual bone. PEEK implants are extremely rigid making their placement difficult but tend to feel more like bone. Porous polyethylene implants have enough rigidity to resist soft tissue deforming forces but enough flexibility to facilitate placement. Its porous surface also allows superficial tissue integration avoiding the capsule formation intrinsic to smooth-surfaced implants. However, soft tissue tends to adhere to the porous surface making implant removal more difficult than the straightforward removal of smooth-surfaced implants (Table 1).

Indications and advantages of CAD/CAM implants

CAD/CAM provides added sophistication to facial implant surgery.[9] It provides 3-dimensional accuracy in implant design and manufacturing specific to the facial skeleton being addressed. This precision potentially minimizes or eliminates limitations intrinsic to the use of "off the shelf" implants and asymmetry of the facial skeleton. CAD/CAM implants are custom-made for the individual patient.

The precise fit of the CAD/CAM implant to the underlying skeletal contour makes for a more predictable result. A fundamental technical problem in placing bilateral implants in similar positions on opposite sides of the face. Remote, inconspicuous incisions routinely provide limited access and therefore limited exposure of the areas to be augmented. Furthermore, the surgeon never has the ability to see the position of both implants in a single view. CAD/CAM implants are made to augment precisely defined areas as well as register onto specific areas of the underlying skeleton, making implant positioning less problematic. They are also designed to avoid any gaps between the posterior surface of the implant and the anterior surface of the skeleton. Gaps are unavoidable when using "off the shelf" implants. These gaps add to the effective projection of the implant. For example, a 2 mm gap beneath a 3 mm implant will result in an unanticipated additive 5 mm in effective projection. An implant designed and manufactured to have its posterior surface mirror that of the underlying skeleton will avoid that unanticipated contour result.

Implant development and design

CT scans are obtained and provide digital imaging and communications in medicine (DICOM) data, which is standard for handling, storing, printing, and transmitting information in medical imaging. These data are then used to create a 3-dimensional image, which is then used for virtual design sessions between surgeons and software engineers to create an implant. This technique is preferred by the authors because it allows millimeter precision of design. The computerized design is then used to manufacture an implant.

Critical in the design process is to recognize the patient's goals. It is useful for the patient to provide photographs of people who have their desired look. Digital manipulation of patient images can also be helpful. The patient should understand that these images are used as guides in the design process and not predictions of the surgical outcome. There is no algorithm that can translate a digitally created change in soft tissue to an implant design that will result in the outer contour

Table 1
Implant material characteristics

	Ease of Placement	Ease of Removal	Rigidity?	Deformed by Soft Tissues?
Silicone Rubber	Easy	Easy	No	Yes
PEEK	Difficult	Difficult	Yes	No
Porous Polyethylene	Moderate	Difficult	Yes	No

change, however. Effective communication between surgeon and patient is invaluable to the design process.

Because the native facial skeleton is not symmetric as previously discussed, implant augmentation will provide a relative symmetry. Chin implants should create symmetry relative to the midline structures—nasal radix, nasal septum, central incisors, and central lip elements. This symmetry should extend from mental foramen to mental foramen (**Fig. 2**).

Lateral to the mental foramen, mandible implants should relate to the width of the upper face. For example, the extent of lateral augmentation of the mandible angles should relate to the lateral orbital rims in the same way. Designing an implant for one side of the face and mirroring it to create an implant for the opposite side will create mandible symmetry only if the mandible and midface were symmetric before augmentation (**Fig. 3**).

Clinical experience has taught the senior author to control the design process. After voicing their goals and preferences, patient participation in the step-by-step design process has proved unrewarding.

Surgery

Preoperative

To optimize oral hygiene, the patient is requested to have a formal dental cleaning the week before surgery and to rinse with chlorhexidine mouthwash for the 3 days before surgery (Video 1). It is our preference to perform chin and mandibular augmentation under general anesthesia (nasotracheal intubation is ideal). This provides a panoramic view of the operative field. The airway is protected while the oral cavity can be optimally prepared. The entire face and oral cavity are prepared with an iodine solution after placement of a throat pack. The operative site is infiltrated with 1/200,000 epinephrine solution to provide hemostasis. Intravenous antibiotics are administered before the incision being made.

Chin incision and dissection

The chin and the anterior mandible are accessed through a submental incision. The midline of the chin is marked on the pogonion as a reference point. Wide subperiosteal dissection is performed. The upper limit of the dissection is the origin of the mentalis muscle, preserving its origin on the bone (**Fig. 4**). Laterally, the mental foramen with its exiting nerve and the inferior border of the mandible body are exposed. Lateral dissection extends approximately 1 cm beyond the area of augmentation. The submental approach and extended dissection avoid damage to the mentalis muscle, allow visualization of the mental nerve, and provide a panoramic view of the complex and varying contours of the mandible to allow precise implant placement. The technique of intraoral placement of chin implants avoids a cutaneous scar but provides limited exposure to the menton and compromises the integrity of the mentalis muscle.

Chin implant positioning and closure

Marking the midline of the pogonion aids in symmetric implant placement. The midline can be marked with a marker, drill hole, or temporary screw. This is useful for implants of any design or material. When using "off the shelf" implants, it may be beneficial to contour prominences on the native mandible to allow better congruence

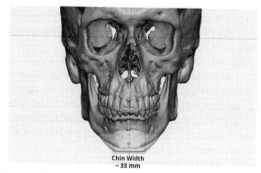

Fig. 2. Chin implant design demonstrates the symmetry relative to midline structures of the face.

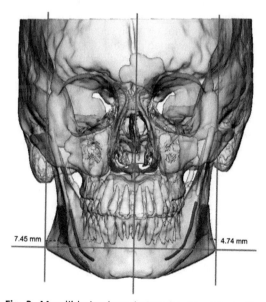

Fig. 3. Mandible implant design should relate to the respective upper face rather than just designing one side and mirroring that onto the contralateral side.

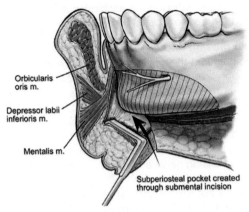

Fig. 4. The submental approach to the chin allows for wide exposure and preservation of the mentalis muscle. *(From* Yaremchuk MJ. Chapter 4: Principles and operative technique for facial skeletal augmentation. In: Yaremchuk, MJ, ed. Atlas of Facial Implants, 2nd ed. Elsevier; 2020:41-49; with permission).

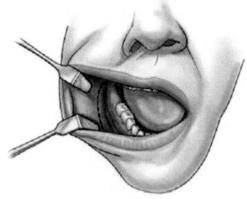

Fig. 5. The intraoral incision made to approach the mandible should be made off of the midline to assure an adequate mucosal cuff for secure coverage. *(From* Yaremchuk MJ. Chapter 4: Principles and operative technique for facial skeletal augmentation. In: Yaremchuk, MJ, ed. Atlas of Facial Implants, 2nd ed. Elsevier; 2020:41-49; with permission).

between the posterior surface of the implant and the mandible surface. Our preference is a two-piece porous polyethylene implant with registration tabs incorporated at the inferior border of the implant. Right and left portions of the implant are placed and positioned. The registration tab dictates lateral positioning. The connecting tab joins the 2 implant segments in the midline and also acts as a hinge to allow the implant to adjust to the unique inclination of the mandible border. It also allows the width of the implant to be varied as dictated by the space between the right and left segments. In most instances, there will be a small gap between the medial aspects of the implant halves, which is not clinically significant. Custom implants are designed for the contours of the chin and provide precise positioning, allowing for the advantages previously stated.

The implant is then fixed to the skeleton with titanium screws. This step helps to avoid any implant movement and to assure that the posterior surface of the implant is congruent with the anterior surface of the skeleton, avoiding undesirable gaps.

After hemostasis is achieved, the incision is closed in layers with reapproximation of the platysma muscle. Secure closure needs to be assured to prevent wound healing complications and subsequent implant exposure and contamination.

Mandible incision and dissection

A generous intraoral mucosal incision is made to expose the ramus and body of the mandible. It is made at least 1 cm above the sulcus on its labial side (**Fig. 5**). The anterior ramus, angle, and body

of the mandible are freed from their soft tissues in the subperiosteal plane. It is important to free both the inferior and posterior borders of the mandible of soft-tissue attachments to allow for accurate implant placement. The use of a J stripper can help facilitate this dissection.

Freeing of the inferior border inevitably violates the pterygomasseteric sling. Care should be taken not to divide the sling as this results in postoperative elevation of the masseter muscle and mid ramus bulging with mastication.[10]

Mandible implant positioning and closure

To assure its desired position and to apply it to the surface of the mandible without gaps, the implant is fixed to the underlying skeleton with titanium screws. A long-guarded drill facilitates screw hole drilling. With vigorous retraction, implant fixation can be done through the intraoral incision without the need for transcutaneous trocar placement. Clamping the implant to the mandible maintains its position during screw fixation. It is important to avoid damage to the inferior alveolar nerve during screw fixation. The nerve usually resides in the center of the ramus.

After hemostasis is appropriate, the wound is irrigated (antibiotic irrigation is a rational adjunct to decrease bacterial contamination in this operation performed through intraoral access). The incision is closed in 2 layers with absorbable sutures. Care is taken to evert the mucosal edges. A small suction drain is placed. We prefer one with a trocar, which allows the skin exit site to be located behind the ear lobule. An elastic tape external compression dressing is used to help apply the soft tissues to the implant and avoid hematoma/seroma formation.

Postoperative care

After surgery, patients spend the night in the surgery center or hospital for monitoring and pain management. The drains are removed on the morning after surgery assuming output is appropriate. They are given an oral prophylactic antibiotic for the first week after surgery as well as an oral narcotic and Tylenol for pain management. They are encouraged to sleep with their head of bed elevated and apply ice liberally for the first 48 to 72 hours after surgery to help reduce swelling. Regarding the intraoral incisions, chlorhexidine mouth rinse is performed 3 times per day for the first week postoperatively. The postoperative diet should include liquids only for the first 2 days after surgery and then advance to soft foods for the next 5 days. They are seen in clinic 1 week after surgery at which time their chin sutures are removed, and their diet is advanced as long as the intraoral incisions are healing well.

Unfavorable Outcomes

Like all other surgeries, esthetic augmentation of the male chin and mandible is not without its possible complications. Generally, specific unfavorable outcomes include infection, hematoma, sensory and motor disturbance, as well as disruption of the pterygomasseteric sling.

In our published series, the infection rate was 2.4% for mandible implant surgery.[11,12] No isolated chin surgeries have suffered infection in the senior author's hands, most likely related to the avoidance of intraoral contamination with the use of submental access. Recognition of and treatment of implant infections must be swift. Antibiotics can suppress implant infections but cannot cure them because of the presence of biofilm formation. Infection ultimately requires implant removal. In the senior author's greater than 25-year experience of facial implants, there have not been any late (greater than 3 months postoperatively) infections without secondary contamination from another procedure such as dental cleaning or filler placement, for example.

Although motor disturbances can be troublesome for patients in the postoperative period, they are temporary. They result most likely from retraction neurapraxia or from merely elevating the soft tissues during dissection. The motor nerves are protected as long as one remains in the subperiosteal plane. Temporary sensory disturbance may also result from intraoperative retraction of the mental nerve, which should always be identified before and after implant placement. Knowledge of the nerve location in the ramus prevents its damage during mandible implant screw fixation. The images provided for CAD/CAM implant design can also provide the precise location of the nerve and its location relative to the implant.

CLINICAL EXAMPLES
Case 1

A 26-year-old man who desired a more masculine chin and mandible. His main esthetic concerns

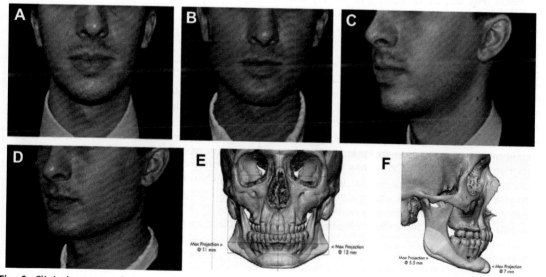

Fig. 6. Clinical case number 1 demonstrates a 26-year-old man who underwent chin and mandible implant augmentation with CAD/CAM implants. His design allowed for increased mandibular angle projection, ramus height, and chin projection per his esthetic goals of a more masculinized look.

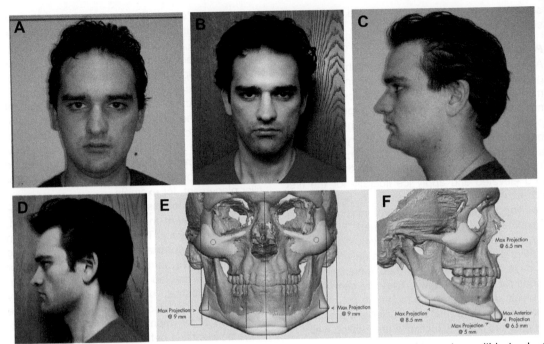

Fig. 7. Clinical case number 2 demonstrates a 28-year-old man who underwent chin and mandible implant augmentation with CAD/CAM implants. His design allowed for increased mandibular angle and chin projection per his esthetic goals of a more masculinized look.

included a lack of mandibular angle definition and a weak chin (**Fig. 6**A, C). Chin and mandible implants were designed with the aid of CAD/CAM to accomplish the goals of increasing angle projection and ramus height as well as giving a stronger and more projected chin (**Fig. 6**E, F). Four years after surgery, the patient was pleased with his result (**Fig. 6**B, D). Of note, after having chin and mandible implant surgery, he also underwent midface augmentation with malar implants, which is also seen in his postoperative photographs.

Case 2

A 28-year-old man who desired a more masculine chin and mandible. His main esthetic concerns included a lack of mandibular angle definition and chin projection (**Fig. 7**A, C). In addition to midface implants, chin and mandibular implants were designed with the aid of CAD/CAM to allow for increased angle and chin projection (**Fig. 7**E, F). Two years after surgery, he was pleased with his result (**Fig. 7**B, D). Of note, he also underwent rhinoplasty at the time of his implant placement.

SUMMARY

The male mandible differs from that of the female in distinct, anatomic ways. These differences play a role in male facial esthetics and can be enhanced by chin and mandible augmentation. Critical components of these procedures include patient evaluation, imaging, preoperative planning, surgery, and postoperative care. If this entire process can be completed in a thoughtful, skillful manner, desirable surgical outcomes can be achieved consistently while minimizing complications.

CLINICS CARE POINTS

- The mandible and chin play a vital role in male esthetics as they contribute to sexual dimorphism.

- The male mandible usually has a longer ramus, more acute gonial angle, wider bigonial distance, and a more squared and projecting chin compared with that of the female.

- Augmentation of the chin and mandible can provide a more esthetic and masculinized appearance.

- Although the chin and mandible can be augmented with osteotomies with bone arrangement and soft tissue augmentation, the authors prefer alloplastic implant augmentation as other methods have undesired downsides.

- CAD/CAM alloplastic implants offer advantages such as balancing natural asymmetries, providing for a more precise surgical placement, and an overall more predictable result compared to "off the shelf" implants.
- When designing CAD/CAM implants for the chin and mandible, they should relate to the upper face structures to provide overall facial balance.
- Surgical placement of alloplastic chin and mandible implants can have predictable and successful outcomes if key surgical maneuvers are applied to the operation.
- Surgical complications such as infection, motor and sensory nerve disturbances, and disruption of the pterygomasseteric sling are associated with implant augmentation of the chin and mandible but can be mitigated with careful patient selection, surgical planning, and precise surgical execution.

DISCLOSURE

The authors have nothing to disclose.

SUPPLEMENTARY DATA

Supplementary data related to this article can be found online at https://doi.org/10.1016/j.cps.2021.12.004.

REFERENCES

1. Fan Y, Penington A, Kilpatrick N, et al. Quantification of mandibular sexual dimorphism during adolescence. J Anat 2019;234(5):709–17.
2. Thiesen G, Gribel BF, Freitas MP. Facial asymmetry: a current review. Dental Press J Orthod 2015;20(6):110–25.
3. Mommaerts MY. The ideal male jaw angle–an Internet survey. J Craniomaxillofac Surg 2016;44(4):381–91.
4. Farkas LGHT, Katic MJ. Anthropometry of the head and face. 2nd edition. New York: Raven Press; 1994.
5. Lee JH, Kaban LB, Yaremchuk MJ. Refining post-orthognathic surgery facial contour with computer-designed/computer-manufactured alloplastic implants. Plast Reconstr Surg 2018;142(3):747–55.
6. Venkatesh E, Elluru SV. Cone beam computed tomography: basics and applications in dentistry. J Istanb Univ Fac Dent 2017;51(3 Suppl 1):S102–21.
7. Yaremchuk MJ. Commentary on: the role of microfat grafting in facial contouring. Aesthet Surg J 2015;35(7):772–3.
8. Pierard-Franchimont C, Goffin V, Pierard GE. Modulation of human stratum corneum properties by salicylic acid and all-trans-retinoic acid. Skin Pharmacol Appl Skin Physiol 1998;11(4–5):266–72.
9. Wagner M, Gander T, Blumer M, et al. [CAD/CAM revolution in craniofacial reconstruction]. Praxis (Bern 1994) 2019;108(5):321–8.
10. Thomas MA, Yaremchuk MJ. Masseter muscle reattachment after mandibular angle surgery. Aesthet Surg J 2009;29(6):473–6.
11. Straughan DM, Yaremchuk MJ. Changing mandible contour using computer designed/computer manufactured (CAD/CAM) alloplastic implants. Aesthet Surg J 2021;41(10):NP1265–75.
12. Yaremchuk MJ, Chang CS, Dayan E, et al. Atlas of facial implants. 2nd edition. Elsevier; 2020.

The Male Abdominoplasty

Michael J. Stein, MD, FRCSC[a,b,*], Alan Matarasso, MD, FACS[a,b]

KEYWORDS

- Male plastic surgery • Male aesthetics • Male abdominoplasty • Male body contouring

KEY POINTS

- Surgeons must consider the unique anatomical differences between men and women presenting for abdominoplasty.
- Male gender is an independent risk factor for complications following abdominal contouring.
- Liposuction, fat grafting, multiple row plications, and strategic scar placement can be used to optimize aesthetic outcomes following male abdominoplasty.

INTRODUCTION

The demand for male body contouring has increased exponentially over the last 2 decades. Although this patient population was historically comprised of overweight men primarily concerned about abdominal girth , it has since become dominated by 2 new patient populations; (1) massive weight loss with mild to moderate adiposity but significant skin excess, (2) young, athletic males seeking to enhance their muscular definition more than can be achieved by exercise alone.

Health, fitness, and sexuality are commonly judged by the appearance of the abdomen, and it is a common source of concern for male patients as they age. As such, abdominal contouring remains one of the most common procedures in plastic surgery, and its popularity continues to increase. In 2016 alone, 181,540 abdominoplasties were performed in the United States, of which 96% were women and 4.4% were men.The number of abdominoplasties increased by 28% from 2012 to 2017.[1] The proportion of men seeking abdominoplasties is projected to increase with an increasing population of patient with massive weight loss[2,3] and emerging minimally invasive technologies, which allow younger patients to enhance their abdominal contour with less downtime.

Since the senior authors review nearly 2 decades ago,[4] few studies have been published about the male abdominoplasty. Surgeons meeting the growing demand must equip themselves with the knowledge of the unique anatomical and technical considerations that make male abdominal contouring different than female. Herein, the authors review the relevant anatomy, technical approach, and postoperative outcomes for the modern male abdominoplasty.

ANATOMICAL DIFFERENCES IN MALE ABDOMINAL ANATOMY

Key anatomic variations in skin, fat, and fascia exist between the male and female abdomen. With respect to skin, although thickness depends on age and genetics, multiple studies have demonstrated increased thickness in men compared to women.[5–7] This may contribute to an increased tendency toward laxity, overstretching, and striations in females versus male patients. Consequently, in non-massive-weight-loss male patients, excessive skin redundancy may require more weight loss to manifest itself.

Significant gender-specific differences exist with respect to abdominal adiposity. Fat distribution is modulated by sex steroids. As such, differences in adipose distribution arise during puberty

[a] Manhattan Eye, Ear and Throat Hospital, 210 E 64th St, New York, NY 10065, USA; [b] Lenox Hill Hospital, 100 E 77th St, New York, NY 10075, USA
* Corresponding author.
E-mail address: mike.stein@nychhc.org

Clin Plastic Surg 49 (2022) 285–291
https://doi.org/10.1016/j.cps.2022.01.002

and persist over the lifetime in men and women. At puberty, there is an increase in body weight, which in men is due to increases in lean mass, whereas in women is due to an increase in fat mass.[8,9] At this time, a classic android and gynoid body habitus begins to develop. Unlike women, men commonly gain their weight centrally, in the abdominal region, and this "apple," android patten of fat distribution has been associated with an increased risk of coronary heart disease.[10] In contrast, the "pear," gynoid pattern of adiposity seen in women has a more gluteofemoral distribution and is thought to confer a lower cardiometabolic risk. Women have a higher percentage of body fat than men, but unlike men, the fat distribution, independent of total body fat, confers protection against metabolic diseases, such as coronary artery disease and diabetes.[11] For men and women with the same body mass index (BMI), women preferentially accumulate more white subcutaneous tissue in the superficial, suprascarpal fat layer.[12] Sex differences in fat distribution relate to cell size. In women, the gluteofemoral adipocytes are larger, and in men, the visceral adipocytes are larger.[13,14] For younger age groups, women also have less intraabdominal fat than men.[15] With increasing age in men, testosterone declines and visceral adiposity increases, contributing to rectus diastasis. In menopausal women, adipose tissue is redistributed to a more android phenotype.[16,17]

Differences in myofascial anatomy also exist. Studies have demonstrated significantly larger rectus abdominus muscles in men compared with women.[18–20] With respect to rectus diastasis, women more commonly present with a lower diastasis leading to a suprapubic bulge, whereas men present with an upper rectus diastasis, leading to a more diffuse and upper abdominal bulge. The cause of rectus diastasis is also unique. One in 3 women experience rectus diastasis 1 year postpartum[21] owing to both physiologic and mechanical weakness at the linea alba. Levels of progesterone, estrogen, relaxin, and corticosterone directly stimulate metalloproteinases, which degrade extracellular matrix, weakening the fascia.[22,23] Abdominal wall compliance also increases 1.5 times by the mechanical stretch of intraabdominal volume during pregnancy, changing the extracellular matrix composition.[24] In men, on the other hand, absolute intraabdominal pressure by visceral obesity and repeated pressure increases during exercise contribute to the rectus diastasis.[25] Some have suggested that certain exercises alone can exacerbate the rectus muscle diastasis.

CONSULTATION WITH THE MALE ABDOMINOPLASTY PATIENT
Patient Presentation

Patient presentation for male abdominoplasties differs significantly from that in females . In the senior authors' last *Clinics of Plastic Surgery* article on the male abdominoplasty in 2004,[4] the common characteristics of the male abdominoplasty were outlined, including older age at presentation, higher presenting weight, and interest in an isolated region. Over the last two decades the demographic of males presenting for abdominal contouring has changed quite significantly. Today, we find men fall into 1 of 3 categories (**Table 1**). The first group of men are often younger , aged 20 to 40 years, and either seek to enhance an existing muscular physique with high-definition liposuction and/or fat grafting, or increase the visibility of their underlying musculature by removing mild infraumbilical skin excess. These patients tend to present with multiple cosmetic concerns and come well read on the multiple procedures that they hope will address it. They have specific goals in mind, and it is not uncommon for them to propose treatments to the plastic surgeons before the surgeon does. It is particularly important to address realistic expectations in this patient population and together come up with a surgical plan that can meet these expectations.

The second group of patients present with a more classic android habitus. They have moderate adiposity and skin excess, rectus diastasis, and a significant contribution of visceral fat. This cohort of patients is at highest risk for dissatisfaction with their final result because of residual protuberance from unaddressed visceral fat. These patients are best pretreated with dieting and exercises to reduce their BMI as much as possible before surgery. Most patients are treated with lipoabdominoplasty, yet higher BMI patients are sometimes better served with a staged procedure, with high volume liposuction performed at the first stage followed by abdominoplasty 3-6 months later.

The final group of patients have undergone massive weight loss following bariatric surgery or by natural means. These patients have a primary concern of excess abdominal skin and suprapubic skin ptosis. These patients are psychologically debilitated by their pannus. They seek to rid themselves of their previous perception of self and live comfortably in their new body. These patients are highly satisfied after surgery, yet their poor skin quality increases risk for wound healing complications and a prolonged postoperative course.

Table 1
Most common male presentation and treatment

Categories	Patient Vignette	Skin	Fat	Fascia	Treatment
I	Young athletic patient seeking to extenuate muscles and get rid of stubborn fat that does not respond to exercise	Minimal laxity	Mild/Moderate	Minimal	Liposuction abdomen/flanks + Superficial liposculpting ("high-definition liposuction") of linea alba, linea semilunaris, and tendinous inscriptions ± Mini-abdominoplasty (if there is focal infraumbilical skin laxity)
II	Middle-aged man with excess skin and fat that does not respond to exercise	Moderate laxity	Moderate/Severe	Lower and upper diastasis	Liposuction abdomen/flanks + Full abdominoplasty + Vertical ± transverse rectus plication (*) *Consider staging*
III	Massive weight loss patient after bariatric surgery or natural weight loss	Severe laxity	Minimal	Variable	Full/extended abdominoplasty (± body lift or fleur de lis if needed) ± Vertical ± transverse rectus plication (only if required)

Physical Examination

Examination of the male abdomen should be performed in standing, sitting, and supine positions. Skin examination should note the presence of scars, bulges, or signs of skin irritation under the pannus. The degree and location of skin excess should be noted, including the presence of suprapubic skin ptosis. Fat examination should note the degree of adiposity (lipodystrophy class 1–3), the location of the adiposity (primarily infraumbilical versus diffuse), and the relative contribution of visceral (intraabdominal) fat. Fascial examination, which should be done in both standing and supine positions, should note the presence of hernias, and the location and approximate distance of the rectus diastasis. When there is clinical suspicion of a hernia, advanced imaging is recommended for further characterization.

Informed Decision Marking and Patient Counseling

Once equipped with the knowledge of the patient's concerns and specific anatomy, the surgeon can now tailor their surgical plan accordingly. The authors' practice is to go through the proposed technique and explain why the chosen technique will specifically address each concern. Local and systemic complications of the procedure are then reviewed, which vary according to the type of procedure being performed. Local complications include infection, hematoma, seroma, wound dehiscence, scar irregularities, umbilical stenosis/necrosis/malposition, skin paresthesia/numbness, contour irregularities, and persistent protuberance from residual intraabdominal fat. Systemic complications include respiratory compromise from elevated intraabdominal pressure, deep vein thrombosis/pulmonary embolism, systemic infection, major wound dehiscence, lidocaine toxicity, visceral injury and death. Surgeons must be reminded that abdominoplasty has a higher systemic complication rate (specifically risk for venous thromboembolism) than any other cosmetic surgery. As such, a detailed plan for perioperative prophylaxis must be considered. A discussion of modifiable risk factors for complications is also prudent, with a thorough preoperative workup advised to identify such factors. The authors recommend at least an electrocardiogram, complete blood count, hemoglobin A_{1c}, nicotine test and nutritional workup (particularly important in massive-weight-loss population for which vitamin and electrolyte deficiencies are common).

The authors then provide the patient with a perioperative instruction packet, which provides information on dressings, showering, drain care, body positioning, pain control, and a timeline for returning to normal activities, such as sexual activity and exercise. They also review an ERAS (enhanced recovery after surgery) protocol , which describes the type of drugs the patient will be prescribed to manage symptoms such as pain, anxiety, nausea/vomiting, and constipation.

ABDOMINOPLASTY TECHNIQUE
Technique Selection

The patient's anatomy dictates the surgical technique (**Table 1**). Group 1 patients have an athletic build and seek to remove modest amounts of fat and/or skin to enhance muscular definition. Many of these patients can be treated with power-assisted liposuction alone. A combination of deep and superficial liposuction (also known as high-definition liposuction) is performed in order to enhance transition zones and natural body concavities and convexities. A pinch test is used as guidance. Superficial liposculpting is performed using a 4-mm basket cannula in the suprascarpal layer along the linea alba, linea semilunaris, and in select cases, over the tendinous inscriptions of the rectus muscle. Fat grafting to the rectus and pectoralis major muscle is also an effective way to further enhance trunk aesthetics. Radiofrequency skin tightening devices are particularly useful in older athletic males who have reduced skin elasticity, and can be used concomitantly with liposuction and/or abdominoplasty. Some group 1 patients have infraumbilical skin laxity that can be addressed surgically. These patients usually need not undergo a full abdominoplasty and are effectively treated with a skin-only mini-abdominoplasty, with skin elevation limited to the infraumbilical region. This procedure is particularly useful in improving the aesthetics of the male umbilicus, as skin resection creates superior hooding.

Group 2 patients present with the classic android, apple-shaped abdomen with moderate amounts of fat and skin excess, varying degrees of intraabdominal fat, and a rectus diastasis. These patients are best treated with a full abdominoplasty or lipoabdominoplasty with or without rectus plication. A frank discussion about the final

contour is critical with these patients, as the amount of intraabdominal fat can significantly limit the final aesthetic. Occasionally, surgeons may also evaluate the need to stage these patients, depending on the amount of liposuction required. In the first stage, aggressive abdominal, flank and/or back liposuction is performed, followed by full abdominoplasty 3-6 months later. The authors have found this technique particularly useful in improving the final aesthetic in higher BMI patients, while improving the safety profile of the operation.

Group 3 patients have classic stigmata of massive weight loss. These include a hanging abdominal pannus with possible underlying skin changes, multiple deflated skin rolls, skin excess laterally (possible circumferentially), and mons ptosis with or without a genital deformity. The patients may or may not have a rectus diastasis and tend not to have a significant degree of intraabdominal fat. These patients are best treated with an abdominoplasty or extended abdominoplasty (270° lift) with conversion to circumferential body lift or fleur-de-lis abdominoplasty if the patient's anatomy would benefit from it. If rectus diastasis is minimal, it is unnecessary to plicate, as it contibutes significantly to the pain profile of the procedure, may increased risk of deep venous thrombosis, and does not improve the final aesthetic.

Abdominal Marking

A vertical line is drawn from the base of the penis to the xiphoid as a reference for the true midline, irrespective of the umbilicus position. Two parallel lines are then marked over the linea semilunaris bilaterally. Incorporating the umbilicus into the midline marking is a common error, increasing the risk for umbilicus malposition, as it is a midline structure in less than 2% of cases.[26] In athletic men undergoing concomitant high-definition liposuction, the authors ask the patient to flex, so the linea semilunaris and tendinous inscriptions of the rectus muscle can be marked statically and dyamically. These reflect the transition zones over which more superficial liposuction is perfromed to enhance muscular defintion. Of note, if performed in the context of an abdominoplasty, the surgeon must medialize their markings in anticipation for the rectus diastasis repair and medialization of the abdominoplasty flap upon closure. Ignoring this will lead to inappropriately placed transition zones upon closure.

The patient then sits, and the extent of the skin creases are marked out laterally with a dot to mark the apex of the skin resection bilaterally. In patient with massive weight loss, these typically extent up to and past the anterior axillary line. If there is significant adiposity laterally and posteriorly, the surgeon should not hesitate to extend circumferentially to prevent dogear formation and poor abdominoplasty flap redraping.

Skin incision placement in men is more flexible than in women and is best designed using the patient's preferred undergarments as reference. Creating a more acute arc is beneficial in women, as it recruits tissue medially and accentuates the waist. This is unnecessary in male patients, so a gentler arc is more appropriate. The lower skin incision is marked while the patient gently grasps and pulls up the skin flap. Superior traction is important, as it accounts for the superior scar migration that occurs following abdominoplasty. It is important to keep the incision parallel and superior to the inguinal ligament to recruit thick tissue for closure and mitigate the risk of injury to the lateral femoral cutaneous nerve of the thigh. The patient is then asked to bend at the waist to mimic bed flexion. A pinch test is then performed to evaluate closure tension and the location of the upper incision.

Abdominal markings in patient with massive weight loss are more challenging. Asymmetric pannus weight makes marking in the standing position difficult. It is easier to mark these patients lying down, where the inferior margin is marked and then one hand retracts the pannus away from the inferolateral markings in the vector that mimics closure tension.

Lipoabdominoplasty Procedure

Liposuction has become a frequently used adjunct to the modern male abdominoplasty. One to two L of tumescent solution is injected to the flanks, upper abdomen, and suprapubic area, keeping in mind the maximal dose of tumescent and epinephrine of 35 to 55 mg/kg and 0.7 mg/kg, respectively. Simultaneous separation and tumescence (SST) uses the Microaire power-assisted liposuction cannula (MicroAire Surgical Instruments LLC, Charlottesville, VA) and a rollerpump to improve the efficiency and safety of infiltration. Liposuction then proceeds in a graded fashion using a 4-mm Mercedes cannula with the knowledge of abdominal flap vascularity.[27] Liposuction is performed deep to prevent contour irregularities, which is the most common complication of abdominal liposuction. Superficial liposuction is then added in select patients with a 4-mm basket cannula to the superficial fat layer, accounting for flap medialization during redraping and closure.

Liposuction instruments are then passed off the field and attention is directed at pannus excision. Markings are verified with a crisscross suture technique at the xiphoid and mons pubis.[28] The umbilicus is incised, and scissors are used to free the umbilical stock from the abdominoplasty flap. The superior incision is then made, and dissection is carried down to the fascia with a 20-blade scalpel. Monopolar cautery is then used to create a narrow tunnel up the xiphoid, preserving perforators from the epigastric arteries medially and intercostal arteries laterally. The anesthesiologist then flexes the table, and the abdominoplasty flap is pulled inferiorly to confirm the previously marked inferior incision. The inferior marking is then made, and pannus is excised from side to side with a 20-blade scalpel while an assistant achieves hemostasis with an insulated forceps and monopolar cautery. Surgeons must make the inferior incision cautiously in the patient with massive weight loss, as the ptotic tissues can distort anatomy and bring critical structures into the plane of excision.

Before diastasis repair, the authors examine for signs of hernia. This is particularly important for the Group 2 male patient, in which hernias are not uncommon. If a hernia is present, it is repaired before midline plication. It is therefore important to discuss and consent for the use of mesh during the preoperative discussion. Small hernias can be closed primarily, whereas larger ones can be closed with an underlay bioabsorbable mesh.

There is no difference in outcomes related to different techniques of rectus diastasis repair.[29] A double-layered closure is performed above and below the umbilicus. The fascial tension is then assessed for the need of additional rows of fascial plications parallel to midline or transversely at the level of the umbilicus. The authors prefer a 0-loop nylon or number 2 PDO quill suture for the running layer. Last, the authors perform transverse abdominus plane blocks with bupivacaine liposome injectable suspension (Exparel), which they find limits (and sometimes eliminates) postoperative narcotic consumption postoperatively.

The authors then tailor tack the flap into place and close with a double layer of barbed sutures (deep layer involves a large bite including Scarpa fascia and dermis with 2-0 PDO Quill, followed by a second subcuticular layer of 3-0 PDO Quill providing closure of the skin.) The umbilicus is then exteriorized through an inverted V incision and inset with 3-0 deep dermal PDS sutures followed by simple interrupted 4-0 nylon suture. Two 14F Jackson Pratt drains are exteriorized and sutured into the incision to decrease scar burden. Alternatively, a newer drain system, such as the Interi internal suction system, can be used. An abdominal binder is sent home with the patient, and they are instructed to start wearing it continuously postoperative day 3 for a duration of 4 weeks.

SURGICAL OUTCOMES FOR MALE ABDOMINOPLASTY

Abdominoplasties in general have among the highest complication profile of any plastic surgery procedure,[30] and male gender has recently been identified as an independent risk factor for complications. Multiple studies support a higher complication rate in men following abdominoplasty. In a study of post bariatric patients, Sirota and colleagues[31] showed that males had over double the complication rate (40.8% vs 20.3%) and that male gender was an independent risk factor for hematoma and seroma formation. These findings echoed a study by Chong and colleagues[32] which illustrated that hematoma and seroma rates were significantly higher in men (14.6% vs 3.5% and 25% vs 13%, respectively). A higher incidence of abdominoplasty complicaitons in males was also noted in retrospective reviews by Momeni[33] and Neaman[34]. In a study of 25,478 abdominoplasties analyzed from the CosmetAssure database, Winocour[30] demonstrated that male gender constituted the largest preoperative risk factor for major complications, with multivariate regressions demonstrating 1.8 times the risk of major complications compared with women undergoing abdominoplasty. A study of 10,473 patients using the American College of Surgeons National Surgical Quality Improvement database by Donato and colleagues[35] similarly reported that male gender was an independent risk factor for any complications (odds ratio, 1.3) and major complications (odds ratio, 1.52), and when panniculectomies were performed, an independent risk fractor for major complications (OR 1.43). Male abdominoplasties also had significantly greater operative times than in females.

SUMMARY

Unique anatomic considerations and cosmetic concerns make the male abdominoplasty different than in females. The male abdominoplasty also is associated with a higher complication profile than in females. Surgeons meeting the increased demand for male body contouring should equip themselves with the knowledge and skills to safely and effectively manage these patients. To optimize results and patient satisfaction, surgeons must risk-stratify patients appropriately, manage modifiable risk factors before operating, and choose the safest and most reliable procedure that will address the patient's specific anatomy.

CLINICS CARE POINTS

- Age, body mass index and male gender are indpendent risk factors for complications following abdominoplasty. Preoperative medical optimizaiton, and managment of modifiable risk factors is important for reducing complications.
- In patients with moderate to severe lipodystrophy and skin excess, consideration of staging liposuction from abdominoplasty reduces surgical risk and improves the aesthetic result.
- High-definition liposuciton and fat grafting are useful adjuncts to the modern male abdominoplasty.

DISCLOSURE

Dr M.J. Stein has no disclosures. Dr A. Matarasso has no disclosures.

REFERENCES

1. Cosmetic surgery national data bank statistics. Aesthet Surg J 2018;38(suppl 3):1–24.
2. Almutairi K, Gusenoff JA, Rubin JP. Body contouring. Plast Reconstr Surg 2016;137:586e–602e.
3. Estimate of bariatric surgery numbers 2011–2016. Available at: https://asmbs.org/%20resources/estimate-of-bariatric-surgery-numbers. Accessed Dec 2020.
4. Matarasso A. The male abdominoplasty. Clin Plast Surg 2004;31(4):555–569, v-vi.
5. Sandby-Møller J, Poulsen T, Wulf HC. Epidermal thickness at different body sites: relationship to age, gender, pigmentation, blood content, skin type and smoking habits. Acta Derm Venereol 2003;83(6):410–3.
6. Firooz A, Rajabi-Estarabadi A, Zartab H, et al. The influence of gender and age on the thickness and echo-density of skin. Skin Res Technol 2017;23(1):13–20.
7. Bailey SH, Oni G, Brown SA, et al. The use of non-invasive instruments in characterizing human facial and abdominal skin. Lasers Surg Med 2012;44(2):131–42.
8. Maynard LM, Wisemandle W, Roche AF, et al. Childhood body composition in relation to body mass index. Pediatrics 2001;107:330–44. https://doi.org/10.1542/peds.107.2.344.
9. Wells JC. Sexual dimorphism of body composition. Best Pract Res Clin Endocrinol Metab 2007;21:415–30. https://doi.org/10.1016/j.beem.2007.04.007.

10. Hsieh SD, Yoshinaga H. Abdominal fat distribution and coronary heart disease risk factors in men-waist/height ratio as a simple and useful predictor. Int J Obes Relat Metab Disord 1995;19(8):585–9.

11. Manolopoulos KN, Karpe F, Frayn KN. Gluteofemoral body fat as a determinant of metabolic health. Int J Obes 2010;34:949–59. https://doi.org/10.1038/ijo.2009.286.

12. Camhi SM, Bray GA, Bouchard C, et al. The relationship of waist circumference and BMI to visceral, subcutaneous, and total body fat: sex and race differences. Obesity (Silver Spring) 2011;19:402–8.

13. Fried SK, Kral JG. Sex differences in regional distribution of fat cell size and lipoprotein lipase activity in morbidly obese patients. Int J Obes 1987;11:129–40.

14. Schreiner PJ, Terry JG, Evans GW, et al. Sex-specific associations of magnetic resonance imaging-derived intra-abdominal and subcutaneous fat areas with conventional anthropometric indices. The Atherosclerosis Risk in Communities Study. Am J Epidemiol 1996;144:335–45.

15. Demerath EW, Sun SS, Rogers N, et al. Anatomical patterning of visceral adipose tissue: race, sex, and age variation. Obesity (Silver Spring) 2007;15:2984–93.

16. Svendsen OL, Hassager C, Christiansen C. Age- and menopause-associated variations in body composition and fat distribution in healthy women as measured by dual-energy X-ray absorptiometry. Metabolism 1995;44:369–73.

17. Toth MJ, Tchernof A, Sites CK, et al. Effect of menopausal status on body composition and abdominal fat distribution. Int J Obes Relat Metab Disord 2000;24:226–31.

18. Tahan N, Khademi-Kalantari K, Mohseni-Bandpei MA, et al. Measurement of superficial and deep abdominal muscle thickness: an ultrasonography study. J Physiol Anthropol 2016;35(1):17.

19. Rho M, Spitznagle T, Van Dillen L, et al. Gender differences on ultrasound imaging of lateral abdominal muscle thickness in asymptomatic adults: a pilot study. PM R 2013;5(5):374–80.

20. Rankin G, Stokes M, Newham DJ. Abdominal muscle size and symmetry in normal subjects. Muscle Nerve 2006;34(3):320–6.

21. Mommers EHH, Ponten JEH, Al Omar AK, et al. The general surgeon's perspective of rectus diastasis. A systematic review of treatment options. Surg Endosc 2017;31(12):4934–49.

22. Hefner L. Maternal adaptations to pregnancy: II. In: The reproductive system at a glance. New York: Wiley-Blackwell; 2010. p. 51.

23. Goldsmith LT, Weiss G. Relaxin in human pregnancy. Ann N Y Acad Sci 2009;1160:130–5.

24. Petrenko AP, Castelo-Branco C, Marshalov DV, et al. Physiology of intra-abdominal volume during pregnancy. J Obstet Gynaecol 2021;41(7). https://doi.org/10.1080/01443615.2020.1820470.

25. Nienhuijs SW, Berkvens EHM, de Vries Reilingh TS, et al. The male rectus diastasis: a different concept? Hernia 2021;25(4):951–6.

26. Rohrich RJ, Sorokin ES, Brown SA, et al. Is the umbilicus truly midline? Clinical and medicolegal implications. Plast Reconstr Surg 2003;112:259–63.

27. Matarasso A, Matarasso DM, Matarasso EJ. Abdominoplasty: classic principles and technique. Clin Plast Surg 2014;41(4):655–72.

28. Matarasso A, Suri S, Stein MJ. Lipoabdominoplasty technique. Plast Aesthet Res 2021;8:57.

29. El Hawary H, Abdelhamid K, Meng F, et al. A comprehensive, evidence-based literature review of the surgical treatment of rectus diastasis. Plast Reconstr Surg 2020;146(5):1151–64.

30. Winocour J, Gupta V, Ramirez JR, et al. Abdominoplasty: risk factors, complication rates, and safety of combined procedures. Plast Reconstr Surg 2015;136(5):597e–606e.

31. Sirota M, Weiss A, Billig A, et al. Abdominoplasty complications - what additional risks do postbariatric patients carry? J Plast Reconstr Aesthet Surg 2021;74(12):3415–20.

32. Chong T, Coon D, Toy J, et al. Body contouring in the male weight loss population: assessing gender as a factor in outcomes. Plast Reconstr Surg 2012;130(2):325e–30e. https://doi.org/10.1097/PRS.0b013e3182589adb.

33. Momeni A, Heior M, Bannasch H, et al. Complications in abdominoplasty: a risk factor analysis. J Plast Reconstr Aesthet Surg 2009;62:1250–4.

34. Neaman KC, Armstrong SD, Baca ME, et al. Outcomes of traditional cosmetic abdominoplasty in a community setting: A retrospective analysis of 1008 patients. Plast Reconstr Surg 2013;131:403e–10e.

35. Donato DP, Simpson AM, Garlick JW, et al. Abdominal contouring and male gender: analysis of complications using the national quality improvement program database. Ann Plast Surg 2019;83(4):481–7.

Contemporary Management of Gynecomastia

Dennis J. Hurwitz, BS, MD[a],*, Armando A. Davila, BS, MD[b,c]

KEYWORDS

- Gynecomastia • Bipolar radiofrequency • Skin tightening • Simon classification of gynecomastia
- Breast ptosis • Liposuction • Boomerang pattern correction of gynecomastia
- Lipoaugmentation of pectoralis muscle

KEY POINTS

- Contemporary management often uses advanced technology of therapeutic ultrasound (VASER) and bipolar radiofrequency (BodyTite and Morpheus8 Body) to reduce morbidity and improve quality of results.
- New skin reduction patterns, such as the boomerang, have reduced skin laxity and the scar burden.
- Masculinization using high-definition liposuction and lipoaugmentation of the pectoralis and deltoid muscles should be offered to appropriate candidates.
- Areolaroplasty reshapes and positions masculine nipple areolas.

 Video content accompanies this article at http://www.plasticsurgery.theclinics.com.

INTRODUCTION/HISTORY/DEFINITIONS/BACKGROUND

Gynecomastia is common benign enlargement of the breast occurring in more than one-third of males.[1] Although the deformity can be fleeting, for those that it persists many are so distressed by poor self-image, depression, anxiety, and social phobia that they seek surgical removal.[2,3] Contemporary management enables smoother correction of deformity with fewer complications and optimally extends to masculinization of the torso with results captured by photodocumentation of chest mobility and dynamics.

Once pathologic increases in systemic estrogen and malignancy are ruled out, plastic surgeons most often operate on idiopathic gynecomastia arising from hormonal imbalance acting on a supersensitive glandular bud or caused by increased endogenous or exogenous administered circulating estrogen or estrogenlike hormones. Associated with a variable degree of fat usually related to body adiposity, glandular gynecomastia varies from slight to considerable firm masses emanating from the areolas. Minimal adiposity gynecomastia, commonly seen in low body mass index (BMI) body builders, is an obliquely oriented, easily isolated firm tube with more mass lateral than medial.[4] Adipose-laden gynecomastia is more spherical with less defined borders. Pseudogynecomastia exhibits sparse gland interspersed in adipose, presenting in obese and older patients, and after massive weight loss. As the breast increases in size so may the areola and breast skin envelope, which needs reduction.

Initially, the magnitude of deformity and its psychosocial impact is assessed. Minimal procedures are easily accepted, whereas complex operations

[a] University of Pittsburgh Medical School, 3109 Forbes Avenue, Suite 500, Pittsburgh, PA 15213, USA;
[b] Hurwitz Center for Plastic Surgery; [c] UNLV School of Medicine, 1701 W Charleston Blvd, Las Vegas, NV 89102, USA
* Corresponding author.
E-mail address: drhurwitz@hurwitzcenter.com

Clin Plastic Surg 49 (2022) 293–305
https://doi.org/10.1016/j.cps.2021.12.003
0094-1298/22/© 2021 Elsevier Inc. All rights reserved.

that may entail significant pain, scarring, and risk must be matched by patient antipathy. Because of its simplicity based on breast size and tissue laxity, the Simon classification[5] was slightly modified to sort out most treatment options (**Table 1**). Grade I is minor enlargement without skin redundancy. Grade IIa is moderate enlargement without skin redundancy. Grade IIb is moderate enlargement with nipple ptosis/deformity and/or minor skin redundancy. Grade IIIa is marked enlargement with nipple ptosis/deformity with skin redundancy. Grade IIIb is marked enlargement with sagging breasts and upper torso skin redundancy. Beyond social inhibitions, if there is a concern of masculinity, we introduce surgical enhancement. Patients either limit their operation to the offending gynecomastia or embrace further surgery for masculinization. As more requests for male body contouring occur, correction of gynecomastia becomes a secondary consideration, so a comprehensive approach is expected.

Because contemporary management offers masculinization of the chest and remaining torso through high-definition liposculpture and excisional surgery, basic masculine aesthetics are introduced. For a more comprehensive 360° torso review that relates sculpture techniques to presenting body type read in this Clinics issue "**The Male Abdominoplasty**," by Michael Stein and Alan Matarasso; Gynecomastia and Male Chest Wall Contouring by Douglas Steinbrech and Eduardo Gonzalez; and "**High-Definition Liposculpture in Men**" by Hoyos and coworkers.[6] For our aesthetic purposes, skin tightly wraps to reveal the broad muscles of a dominant upper body. A barrel-like rib cage is draped by large, thick, and flat Pectoralis Major, Trapezius, and Latissimus Dorsi muscles. The lateral edges of these muscles are defined with further pectoral prominence of its midportion and along the lateral border of the sternum. Broad shoulders extend further by apple-like deltoids. Anterior chest definition is completed with inferior Pectoralis fullness superior to a short horizontal flattened adherence near the fifth rib.

The aesthetic goals of the treatment of gynecomastia has traditionally been limited to near total glandular resection, smooth contour transition to surrounding subcutaneous tissue, and removal of loose skin, leaving proper nipple areolar complex (NAC) position and shape with as few scars as possible. Because of pubescent onset of gynecomastia and potential for gender ambiguity this focused approach may leave a sense of inadequate masculinity. With the advent of improved, reliable, and safe male-specific operations and liposculpture, selected patients should be offered more thorough body contouring surgery. Hence, in addition to obliteration of the gynecomastia, contemporary management offers tight-skinned upper torso that reflects underlying musculature enhanced by perimeter etching and lipoaugmentation that should extend surgically throughout the torso.[7] Critically, the inframammary fold (IMF), which lies about one interspace below the inferior pectoral border, needs to be obliterated. Conversely, accentuating the IMF through an inferior chest transverse excision is disastrously feminizing. Although not always obvious standing erect, when leaning residual lax skin drapes over the constructed IMF, revealing a deflated but still sagging breast. The ideal nipple projects several millimeters and is surrounded by a flat, transversely oriented 1.5 to 2.0 cm × 2.5 to 3.0 cm oval areola, lying several centimeters medial and superior to the inferior/lateral junction of the Pectoralis Major muscle. Repositioning of a ptotic nipple relates to dynamic Pectoralis Major muscles rather than skeletal landmarks or absolute numbers or ratios. Large, rounded, and protruding areolas need reshaping.

Ignored by most plastic surgeons, but not by the body-conscious patient, are dynamic shape changes of the chest as the Pectoralis Major

Table 1
Treatment options for Simon grade deformity

Grade	Pull Through	VASERlipo	BodyTite	Pectoralis Lipoaugmentation	Boomerang Pattern	J-Torsoplasty/ Hockey Stick	Double Mastectomy with Free NAC Graft
I	X						
IIa	X	X		X			
IIb	X	X	X	X	X		
IIIa		X	X	X	X	X	
IIIb		X		X	X	X	X

morphs from relaxation to full contraction, and with different positions of the arms and body. Demonstrating and photographing these subtle relationships are appreciated by the patient, aid in treatment planning, and thoroughly document outcomes. For example, Case 1 is a 49-year-old man with BMI of 26, moderate enlargement, nipple ptosis, and moderate skin redundancy, grade IIb (**Figs. 1** and **2**). Descending deep and inferior to the NAC, relaxed Pectoralis muscles are visually inseparable from the gynecomastia (see **Fig 1**, top). The contracted Pectoralis major rises and bulges toward the clavicles isolating the periareolar rounded gynecomastia (see **Fig 1**, bottom). Raising the arms stretches, elevates, and flattens the Pectoralis muscle to isolate the breast mound visually and palpably (**Fig 2**, left). On leaning, the gland with excess skin that is loosely adherent to the Pectoralis muscle disturbingly droops (see **Fig 2**, left). Because the contracted Pectoralis muscle or raised arms leaves no muscle fill deep and inferior to the areola, gynecomastia correction

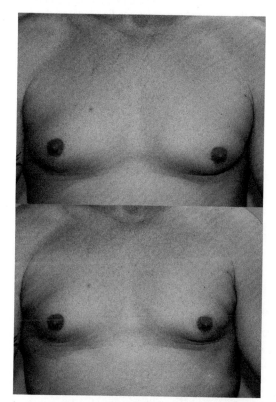

Fig. 1. Grade IIb gynecomastia in a 45-year-old 6-ft, 3-in 200-lb man. Frontal view. (*Top*) With pectoralis muscle relaxed the postareolar skin and inferior is smoothly filled with breast and muscle. The midpectoralis has slight convexity. (*Bottom*) With pectoralis contracted, the muscle is elevated to broadly round the midchest, leaving only rounded and more defined gynecomastia fullness behind and inferior to NAC.

should be planned accordingly. For a thorough visual appraisal of results, comprehensive photographic documentation of gynecomastia and its treatment should include arms to the side, contracted Pectoralis muscle, extended arms, and diving position. Using VASERlipo (Solta Medical, Bothell, WA) and BodyTite (InMode, Irving, CA) (discussed later), total correction is documented in these various positions (**Figs. 3** and **4**).

TECHNIQUES

Improved technology, skin resection patterns, and masculinization procedures have evolved since the senior author (DJH) started practice in 1977. In lean bodybuilding males, transareolar excision of gynecomastia followed by internal suture plication to avoid hematoma has not changed since published in 1989 by Aiache.[8] When there is excess adipose, a broad expanse of full-thickness liposuction has resulted in less bleeding, smoother contours, and limited skin contraction.[9] Since the late 1990s, ultrasonic-assisted lipoplasty partial evacuation of gynecomastia and surrounding excess adipose has been an essential technology for correction of gynecomastia.[10] VASER, a third-generation ultrasonic technology, is popular with surgeons performing high-definition liposuction, citing lower blood loss and smoother results.[6,7,11,12] Compared with traditional and power-assisted lipoplasty, VASERlipo with VenTx cannula aspiration removes more adipose cells with less disruption of neurovasculature and supporting connective tissue, thereby optimizing safety and innate skin shrinkage. Typically, ultrasonic assisted lipoplasty (UAL) leaves behind a reduced mass of firm glandular tissue, expediting less extensive, near bloodless pull-through excision through an infra-areolar incision.[13] Perimeter liposuction tapers the contour leaving behind broad connective tissue adherences from dermis to the muscular facia to abet large area contraction, while reducing the incidence of hematomas or seromas.

Nevertheless, critics lump VASER with other high-energy delivery systems, such as laserlipo causing skin contraction through thermal injury.[14] To the contrary, proper use of VASER causes no destructive heat.[15] Use room temperature infusion fluid. Inject more than the amount of anticipated extraction. Use VASER vibratory mode at 80% or less, with constant probe motion. Continuous mode is reserved for deep fat fragmentation. Withdraw the probe on gaining minimal resistance, which is less than a minute for each anticipated 100 mL of extraction. Skin shrinkage follows preservation of elastic connective tissue and dermis,

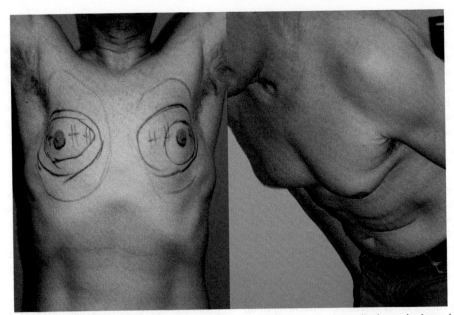

Fig. 2. Arm extension and leaning views of patient in **Fig. 1**. (*Left*) Raising the arms displaces the lateral pectoralis muscle superomedial to isolate the gynecomastia, which is encircled in *blue*. The *small blue circle* represents the perimeter of the palpable gynecomastia. The *outer blue circle* is the extent of excess fat needing tapered removal with VASERlipo. The *green circle* encompasses the area for application of 30 kJ with surface temperature 40°C and deep 70°C bipolar frequency BodyTite. (*Right*) Left anterior oblique diving view shows hanging lax skin.

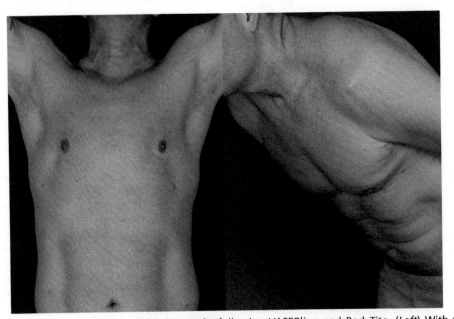

Fig. 3. The same patient in **Figs. 1** and **2**, 7 months following VASERlipo and BodyTite. (*Left*) With the arms extended the pectoralis raises above the areolas revealing no residual breast gland. (*Right*) As the patient leans the areola and inferior is filled with muscle but the skin does not sag.

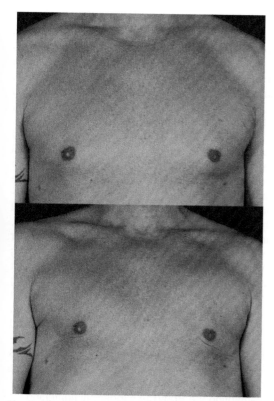

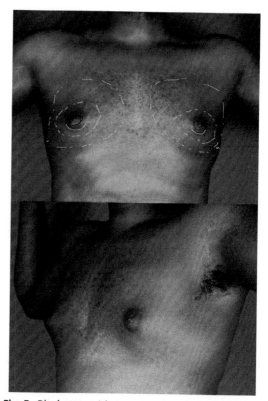

Fig. 4. The same patient in **Figs. 1** and **2**. (*Top*) Seven months postoperatively without gynecomastia his relaxed pectoralis muscle is uniformly flat and fills the lateral and inferior muscle margins. (*Bottom*) With full contraction the pectoralis bulges like an oblique football, to empty the NAC, which slightly tilts inward.

Fig. 5. Black man with preoperative grade IIa gynecomastia. The preoperative markings are *yellow* for infra-areolar incision, *blue* for the areolarplasty, *green* for extent of the palpable gynecomastia, and *white* for the extent of the UAL.

which is free to shorten after evacuation of superficial fat. To verify that high temperature is not part of VASERlipo, subcutaneous tissue temperature was taken in four abdominal locations after completing each VASERlipo stage. Initial tissue temperature averaged 37°C, after room temperature saline infusion temperature averaged 35°C, after VASER application temperature averaged 40°C, and after BodyTite temperature was as high as the goal of 70°C. When the aim is to remove as much fibroglandular tissue as possible, VASER has a gynecomastia probe or consider LySonix 3000 with inline suction (Byron Mentor, Irvine, CA). Using the golf tee tip and power at six, energy is focused on the end, and leads to greater plow through glandular and dense fibrofatty tissue. Emulsified fat streams through the inline probe and tubing.

Grade IIa is a common presentation, which is treated expeditiously under local anesthesia with low risk. Case 2 is a 32-year-old muscular man, BMI of 29.4, with grade IIa gynecomastia, which

appeared during adolescence and enlarged with growth and excess weight gain (**Fig. 5**). He dislikes the feminine mass of breast and the enlarged and hemispherical NACs. Both athletic and a body builder, he will not expose his chest in public. A large mass of firm fat has a central core of firm nodular tissue. Video 1 shows the planning and correction of gynecomastia using LySonix UAL over the entire chest and a pull through of residual gland under regional xylocaine infiltration and oral sedation. UAL removed 180 mL of emulsion and left a honeycomb pattern of dense connective tissue and reduced mass of glandular tissue that was bloodlessly excised (**Fig. 6**). His enlarged and rounded NACs, on superior pedicles, are reduced and shaped to horizontal ellipses allowing for barbed suture purse string closure to flat horizontal ellipses (**Fig. 7**). These high-tech sutures, now with 12 barbs to a centimeter, are sinched after every two bites. Thus, the suture holds alignment and elliptical form. Not pulling the ends of a smooth suture that avoids a purse string new circular areola. This rim excision of NAC skin is called an areolaroplasty, which slightly tightens chest

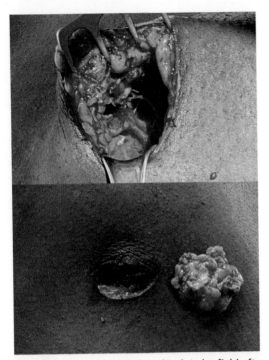

Fig. 6. Gynecomastia resection. (*Top*) A dry field after UAL, which leaves a dense honeycomb patterned of connective tissue with most of the residual gynecomastia under the rake retractor. (*Bottom*) The small residual gland resection lies next to the NAC.

skin and is adapted to treat tuberous breast and NAC hernia deformity. The 4-month result shows a complication-free and aesthetically pleasing correction (**Fig. 8**).

The grade IIb patient needs skin tightening through either broad skin excisions or through application of bipolar radiofrequency. Usually, first-stage VASER emulsification is followed by BodyTite and Morpheus8 Body (InMode, Irvine, CA) to reduce skin laxity and breast ptosis (see Case 1, **Figs 1-4**). Because VASER mode leaves intact most of the subcutaneous tissue supporting the connective network, which is the target for the radiofrequency energy, we usually complete fat emulsification before starting BodyTite. BodyTite uses a bipolar handpiece connected to a radiofrequency energy generating console.[16–18] A 3-mm diameter solid, slightly malleable 20-cm-long probe with a protective end plastic hub is inserted under the dermis through a stab wound incision. On the pull-back continuous probe focused radiofrequency energy is directed to the coupled 3-cm receiving disk gliding on the skin surface. Emanating continuous preset magnitude of radiofrequency energy, the probe slowly traverses, like one would a VASER probe, through all layers of saline-infused subcutaneous tissue, emanating a

steady cadence of clangs. As the preset temperatures are reached, the clangs double sound and on reaching the preset temperatures of around 40°C for the surface and 70°C internal there is a triple clang signaling stoppage of power. At that time, a palm-sized region has absorbed from 5 to 7 kJ. Up to 20% tissue contraction is visualized. If not, then the treatment may be repeated after cooling. It is imperative to heat the tissues adequately and uniformly as indicated by setting 40°C external and 70°C internal limits. If internal limits are reached prematurely before external, slower motion of the probe may be required. Likewise, reaching external temperatures before proper internal heating may be a result of poor tumescent cooling, inappropriate depth of the probe or need faster motion of the probe. Early postoperative swelling masks the collagen injury and shortening, but with proper splinting and maturation of healing the final roughly 30% contracted state is evident 6 to 12 months later as seen in Case 1. Wrinkled skin is worsened by subdermal tightening and needs a multilayered approach with surface bipolar frequency microneedling using Morpheus8 Body, which can now penetrate the surface 7 mm. This results in dermal level smoothing, complementing the BodyTite subdermal tightening.

For most grade III deformity, innovative patterns for large skin resections have been effective and leave more acceptable scars and contours than the simple amputation style transverse excision. With the boomerang mastopexy, the lateral torso hockey stick, and the double mastectomy incision pattern one may apply similar base aesthetic principles. These patterns focus on obviating the IMF as critical and avoiding the incision line along the existing IMF, which feminizes the torso and leaves the scar in the incorrect shadows of the chest. The popularity of bariatric surgery has greatly increased demand for correction of gynecomastia in the context of coordinated total body contouring.[19,20] Massive weight loss can result in severely ptotic breasts with considerable residual gland and skin laxity that includes the entire torso. Combining the upper chest procedures with a J-torsoplasty, we then rely on oblique flankplasty with lipoabdominoplasty to treat the lower body.[21]

DISCUSSION

Since 2017, one or more combination of the following nine procedures corrects gynecomastia and further enhances masculinity:

1. Infra-areolar glandular excision
2. Barbed sutured areolarplasty
3. Inframammary fold disruption

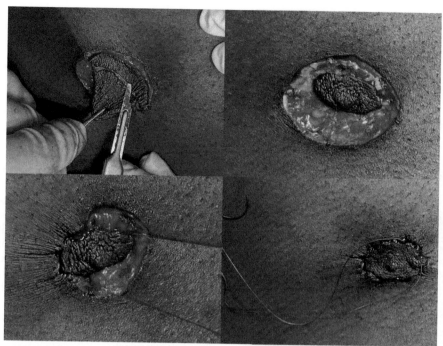

Fig. 7. An areolaroplasty on an oversized hemispherical areola of patient in **Fig. 5**. Access to resection of gyneco-mastia is through infra-areolar incision. (*Top left*) After the inferior excess areola is excised, the superior excess is being deepithelialized. (*Top right*) An elliptical NAC is vascularized by a superiorly based deepithelialized flap. (*Bottom left*) Double armed 3–0 Monoderm barbed suture securely approximates the first third of the skin closure in an elliptical pattern by placing larer bites through the outer rim. (*Bottom right*) The completed closure leaves a flat horizontally oriented elliptical NAC.

4. UAL ablation and adipose evacuation of the chest
5. VASERlipo of the torso with muscular definition
6. Bipolar radiofrequency tissue tightening
7. Boomerang pattern excision, inferior pedicle areolaroplasty with/without J-torsoplasty
8. Lateral torso hockey stick with or without double incision mastectomy with pedicled or free graft areolaroplasty
9. Lipoaugmentation of the pectoralis and deltoid muscles

These therapeutic options are arrayed across the modified Simon classification (see **Table 1**).

Glandular excision for grades I and IIa is typically performed through an infra-areolar incision.[8,22] Adipose free gynecomastia is usually slightly tender, but intermittent disturbing pain and tenderness can occur. Direct excision for grade I gynecomastia removes the tumor and relieves pain. A thin disk of 1 to 1.5 cm of subareolar gland is retained to avoid areolar saucer cup depression. For grade IIa with increased adiposity, the sausage-like firm mass and surrounding excess subcutaneous tissue used to be directly excised with tapering to the perimeter.[4,8] Because

confined by a 3-cm incision, hematoma, seroma, delayed healing, and contour deformity were common, as was early postoperative surgical drainage of hematoma and seromas and secondary correction. Several decades ago, the introduction of UAL has reduced those sequelae. Case 2 demonstrates our current approach for grade IIa associated with chest adiposity.

The skin tightening role of bipolar radiofrequency was demonstrated in Case 1. Case 3 has larger grade IIb gynecomastia with a well-defined IMF in a 190-lb 29 year old, who lost 40 lb (**Figs. 9** left and **10** top). Defined IMFs have a condensation of fibrous adherences between the dermis and the muscular fascia through a reduced adipose area along the inferior portion of the breast. The IMF tends to lie about the sixth rib, whereas the adherences of skin in the male relate to the inferior and lateral borders of the pectoralis muscle, which are one interspace higher. To obtain that aesthetics, the fold is obliterated by stretching and advancing the tissues as happens with lipoabdominoplasty. Also, UAL and BodyTite disrupt the IMF but the fold can also be released directly. VASERlipo of the breasts is followed by superior areolar incision pull through of residual gland and

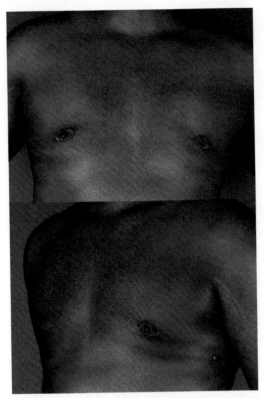

Fig. 8. Black man with grade IIa gynecomastia 4 months after UAL, pull through excision, and elliptical areolaroplasty with complete correction of his feminizing deformity.

30-kJ BodyTite treatment per breast. Nine months later the gynecomastia, its associate adiposity, defined IMF, and skin laxity have been corrected with minimal scars (see **Figs. 9** right, 11 bottom).

Improper use of either VASER or BodyTite can cause subdermal thermal injury leading to hyperpigmentation or hypertrophic scar. But because of the high degree of thermal energy produced during BodyTite, these injuries tend to be more severe. Emit the energy only on the pull back, and take care to avoid excessive pressure causing bowing of the probe or overheating about the entry site. In Case 4, overheated dermis at the entry site resulted in a broad streak of periareolar pigmentation and a depressed skin (**Fig. 11**). Secondary direct excision of the hyperpigmented skin left an acceptable appearance. Scattered abdominal hyperpigmentation caused by tape and dressings is indicative of his hypersensitive hyperpigmentation response even to external pressure. His horizontal elliptical areolas are a result of an barbed sutured areolarplasty. This single-stage total body lift includes   oblique   flankplasty   with lipoabdominoplasty.

Dozens of cases of gynecomastia have been treated with BodyTite. There have been no seromas, skin necrosis, neuropathy, or infections. All patients recognized skin tightening but some had hoped for more and some may obtain further improvement with repeat in-office treatment.

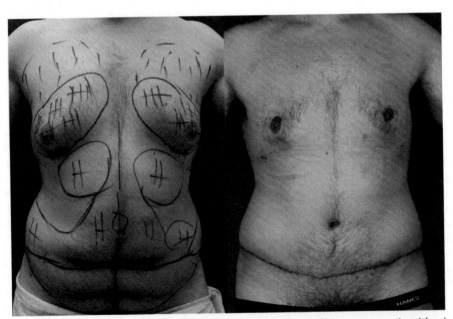

Fig. 9. Case 3. A 190-lb 29 year old with 40-lb weight loss seeks correction of his gynecomastia with minimal scars and abdominoplasty, and VASERlipo of the flanks. (*Left*) Preoperative markings for his 1350-mL VASERlipo evacuation of the breasts followed by 30-kJ BodyTite and lipoabdominoplasty/VASERlipo of the flanks. (*Right*) The 10-month result has correction of his gynecomastia, excellent torso contours, and no loose skin.

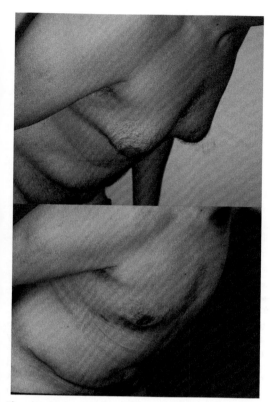

Fig. 10. Right anterior oblique diving view before (*top*) and 10 months after (*bottom*) in the patient presented in **Fig. 9**. The sagging breasts are absent and the inferior chest fold now relates to the lower border of the pectoralis muscle.

Patients with several hundred pounds of weight loss and advanced age do not adequately respond to BodyTite. A cardiac pacemaker is a contraindication.

Grade III demands broad patterns of skin resection. For this grade, a transverse mastectomy, with either a deepithelialized inferior pedicle for the NAC with a free nipple graft or inferior pedicle, is the customary procedure.[19] The unsightly long inferior scar tends to accentuate the IMF and when an inferior deepithelialized pedicle is used, there is undesirable infra-areolar fullness.

For older men with involutional gynecomastia, skin laxity, and mild nipple ptosis, a lateral chest hockey stick skin excision toward the axilla tightens the skin and rests in the shadow of the lateral pectoral border. Case 5 is a 68-year-old man with a lateral torsoplasty (**Fig. 12**). Lateral deviation of the areola is countered with a medial crescent advancement of the NAC. Some residual skin laxity is expected, but a long anterior chest scar is avoided.

Boomerang pattern correction of gynecomastia corrects the nipple ptosis, glandular hypertrophy, and excess anterolateral chest skin.[20,23] The procedure removes two unequal obliquely oriented ellipses, that superiorly straddle the areolas, resembling an Australian boomerang. Considerable tissue in the horizontal and vertical planes is removed with the long closure across the chest visually interrupted by the areola. For grade IIIb, which exhibits circumferential upper body skin laxity, the boomerang pattern was originally extended by a transverse posterior upper body lift. For the past 10 years, the back scar has been avoided and the anterior chest skin further tightened by a lateral thoracic J-torsoplasty.[24] The Boomerang excision pattern for gynecomastia includes extensive indirect inferior chest undermining of the skin to disrupt the IMF.

Case 6 is a 6-ft, 1-in, 240-lb man who sought correction of grade IIIb gynecomastia. However, he was receptive to total body masculinization via a TULUA[25] (transverse plication, no undermining, full liposuction, neoumbilicoplasty, and low transverse abdominal scar) with etching liposuction, oblique flankplasties, and boomerang pattern correction of gynecomastia with J-torsoplasty and muscular lipoaugmentation (**Figs. 13–15**, Video 2). The boomerang design leaves the NAC attached atop a triangular, broad-based, nondeepithelialized inferior pedicle, which is defatted and indirectly undermined through VASERlipo. A C-shaped extension of the lateral chest elliptical excisions then extends vertically to the axilla, allowing the J-torsoplasty to further tighten the midback and the chest. The scar lies under the relaxed arm and not across the back.

The operation began prone with simultaneous oblique flankplasties and fat harvested from the excision sites (Video 3). On turning supine three operations were performed simultaneously: each boomerang/J-torsoplasty combination and the minimally undermined TULUA with infraumbilical transverse plication followed by VASERlipo etching of the rectus abdominus.

The resection of gynecomastia and excess skin over the Pectoralis muscle was essentially bloodless but not so with the lateral chest wall, which is expeditious after early identification of Latissimus Dorsi muscle. Then the dissection proceeds anteriorly across the serratus muscle. On elevation of the descended NAC to its proper location, inferior pole breast and upper abdominal skin laxity are corrected. The weight of tissue removal was 4900 g. With broad exposure of the Pectoralis Major muscles precise injection of processed liposuction fat is placed submuscular and intramuscular. His 300-mL augmentation enhances the muscles and further reduces skin laxity. Closure with #1 barbed Quill sutures of the different length limbs

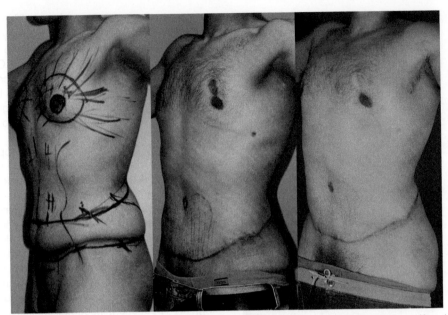

Fig. 11. Case 4. Grade IIb gynecomastia in a 23-year-old patient with massive weight loss who suffered hyperpigmentation injury secondary to excess radiofrequency heat to the dermis. (*Left*) Marking for lipoabdominoplasty with oblique flankplasty, barbed suture areolaroplasty, with glandular pull through after VASERlipo and BodyTite of the anterior chest. (*Middle*) Eighteen months postoperative with scattered hyperpigmentation of scars and from binder pressure on tubing. (*Right*) Six months after excision of depressed hyperpigmentation scar of left chest. The gynecomastia has been correct with well-shaped and positioned NACs. Torso contours and skin tension are excellent.

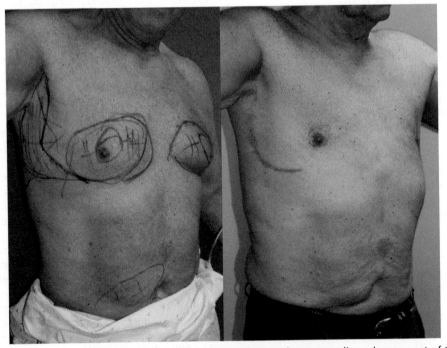

Fig. 12. Combination of a hockey stick–shaped lateral torsoplasty and anteromedian advancement of the nipple areolar complex in a 64-year-old man with 20-lb weight loss leaving grade IIb gynecomastia (*left*). Correction of gynecomastia and loose skin with a lateral chest and periareolar scars (*right*).

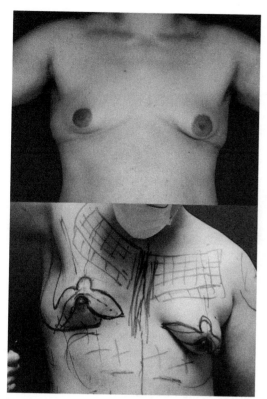

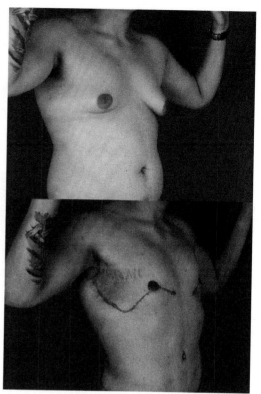

Fig. 13. A recent total body lift in a 33-year-old man who had the boomerang correction of gynecomastia with J-torsoplasty and lipoabdominoplasty with Oblique Flankplasty videotaped (Videos 2 and 3). (*Upper*) The preoperative condition and (*Lower*) marked for surgery frontal views show the deformity and the operative plan. The circumareolar Boomerang pattern is continuous with the J Torsoplasty, along with VASERlipo of the abdomen and lipoaugmentation of the Pectoralis and Deltoid muscles. The simultaneous two-team approach was under the direction of the senior author, who performed the upper body surgery while the junior author (DAA) performed the lower body oblique flankplasty and lipoabdominoplasty (not seen). (*Top*) Images are the frontal and right anterior oblique preoperative images. (*Bottom*) Completed preoperative surgical markings are shown. Video 2 shows the order of the markings for boomerang pattern with J-torsoplasty and the pectoralis muscle grafting. Video 3 shows a highly edited 4-hour operation. The superior incision first, for the proper location of the NAC, particularly when a concomitant abdominoplasty is done. The precise width of elliptical resection is made after the abdominoplasty closure is started. Then after indirect undermining of the lower chest with a LaRoe dissector (ASSI.com), areola is advanced up to the upper markings and they are adjusted as needed for the optional tension at closure. Once the boomerang has been closed, the width of the lateral chest skin excision of the J-torsoplasty is precisely measure and completed.

Fig. 14. A recent total body lift in a 33-year-old man who had the boomerang correction of gynecomastia with J-torsoplasty videotaped along with Oblique Fankplasty and TULUA . (**Fig. 13**, Videos 2 and 3). *Upper* image is the right anterior oblique preoperation. The *lower* right oblique shows the result 3 months postoperative, before he started his work-out routine.

is a challenge in wound edge justification. Because of the structural quality of chest wall skin, when the closure is tight, there is no delayed laxity as is seen commonly in the lower torso.

With tissue resections going in a variety of directions, when combined with lower body lift surgery the operation is technically demanding but usually works out that the tissue contours are all smooth and tight.[26,27] There have been a few instances of unevenness requiring further liposuction or lipoaugmentation. Generally, early boomerang scars are pigmented and thick, but fade and thin over several years. While performing more than 30 cases, only one entire nipple areolar complex sustained necrosis because of overthinning. The limitation of the boomerang pattern is that if after raising the NAC there is still too much infraareolar skin some lax excess skin needs to be removed later. Otherwise in cases of severe hypertrophy and laxity an operation with a free nipple graft is needed. Evolutions of transverse excisions

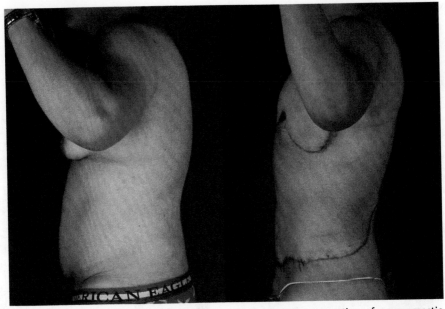

Fig. 15. A recent total body lift in a 33-year-old man had the boomerang correction of gynecomastia with J-tor-soplasty videotaped (**Figs 13, 14** and Videos 2 and 3). Left lateral views show the deformities (*Left*) and the three month result that includes flankplasty with lipoabdominoplasty (*Right*).

have emphasized a dual incision approach, which complements the same principles we have stated previously: first addressing the upper chest laxity with an incision designed to rest at the inferior pectoral border, and the secondary inferior incision designed to match. Destruction of the connective bands at the IMF are once again essential to this technique, and J shaped extension can take up additional lateral laxity.

SUMMARY

We find healthy young men with minimal glandular tissue (grade I, IIa) respond incredibly well with no residual deformity through either transareolar direct excision and/or UAL. For patients grade IIb up to IIIa, VASERlipo is followed by BodyTite. If needed, glandular pull through excision completes the correction with or without barbed sutured areolarplasty. More severe cases require excisional skin tightening, with a variety of patterns suitable for each patient depending on their deformity. What sets plastic surgeons apart is recognizing, predicting, and executing tissue reconstructive procedures assisted by new technology and innovated techniques leaving a proper sculptured result under moderate skin tension that heals rapidly with the fewest and thinnest scars possible rather than a one-size-fits-all approach.

CLINICS CARE POINTS

- Traditional glandular excision of gynecomastia for grades I and IIa is typically performed through infra-areolar incision after UAL of the soft tissues across the chest.

- With skin laxity or following extensive volume aspiration through liposuction, chest skin tightening and elevation of the nipple are performed in selected cases by bipolar radiofrequency technology.

- New excision patterns, such as the boomerang and J-torsoplasty, most aesthetically correct grade III gynecomastia.

- Comprehensive approach to gynecomastia considers surgical masculinization of the entire torso.

DISCLOSURE

Dr D.J. Hurwitz receives annual royalties from Springer Verlag for 2016 textbook, *Comprehensive Management of Body Contouring Surgery*; and received stock options in InMode, Yoakum, Israel for 2 years of clinical studies performed for Food and Drug Administration oversight of bipolar radiofrequency instrument called BodyTite for the reduction of skin laxity. Dr A.A. Davila has no potential conflicts to disclose.

SUPPLEMENTARY DATA

Supplementary data to this article are found online at https://doi.org/10.1016/j.cps.2021.12.003.

REFERENCES

1. Nuttall FQ. Gynecomastia as a physical finding in normal men. J Clin Endocrinol Metab 1979;48(2): 338–40.
2. Kinsella C Jr, Landfair A, Rottgers SA, et al. The psychological burden of idiopathic adolescent gynecomastia. Plast Reconstr Surg 2012;129(1):1–7.
3. Nuzzi LC, Cerrato FE, Erickson CR, et al. Psychosocial impact of adolescent gynecomastia: a prospective case–control study. Plast Reconstr Surg 2013; 131(4):890–6.
4. Blau M, Hazani R. Correction of gynecomastia in body builders and patients with good physique. Plast Reconstruc Surg 2015;135:425–32.
5. Simon BE, Hoffman S, Kahn S. Classification, and surgical correction of gynecomastia. Plast Reconstr Surg 1973;51:48–52.
6. Hoyos AE, Perez ME, Domínguez-Millán R. Gynecomastia treatment through open resection and pectoral high-definition liposculpture. Plast Recons Surg 2021;5(147):1072–83.
8. Aiache A. Surgical treatment of gynecomastia in the body builder. Plast Recon Surg 1989;83(1):61–6.
7. Hoyos AE, Perez ME, Dominquez-Millan R. Variable sculpting in dynamic definition Body contouring: procedure selection and management algorithm. Aesth Plast Surg 2021;41(3):318–32.
9. Rosenberg GJ. Gynecomastia: suction lipectomy as a contemporary solution. Plast Reconstr Surg 1987; 80(3):379–86.
10. Rohrich RJ, Ha RY, Kenkel JM, et al. Classification and management of gynecomastia: defining the role of ultrasound-assisted liposuction. Plast Reconstr Surg 2003;111(2):909–23.
11. Hoyos A, Millard J. VASER-assisted high definition liposculpture. Aesth Surg J 2007;27(6):594–604.
12. Hoyos AE, Guarin DE. Chapter 13 high-definition body contouring using VASER-assisted liposuction. In: Garcia O, editor. Ultrasonic assisted lipoplasty: current concepts and techniques. Springer Nature; 2020. p. 203–11.
13. Hammond DC. Surgical correction of gynecomastia. Plast Reconstr Surg 2009;124(1 Suppl):61e–8e.
14. Wall SH, Claiborne JR. Discussion, a report of 736 high definition of lipoabdominoplasties performed in conjunction circumferential VASER liposuction. Plast Recon Surg 2018;28(142):676–8.
15. Hurwitz DJ. Chapter 12 ultrasound-assisted liposuction in the massive weight loss patient. In: Garcia O, editor. Ultrasonic assisted lipoplasty: current concepts and techniques. Springer Nature; 2020. p. 189–202.
16. Hurwitz DJ, Smith D. Treatment of overweight patients by radiofrequency assisted liposuction (RFAL) for aesthetic reshaping and skin tightening. Aesth Plast Surg 2011;36(1):62–71.
17. Theodorou SJ, Del Vecchio D, Chia CT. Soft tissue contraction in body contouring with radiofrequency-assisted liposuction: a treatment gap solution. Aesth Surg J 2018;38(S2):S74–83.
18. Hurwitz DJ, Wright L. Noninvasive abdominoplasty in abdominoplasty edited by Matarasso A, Zins JE. Clin Plast Surg 2020;47:379–88.
19. Gusenoff JA, Coon D, Rubin JP. Pseudo gynecomastia after massive weight loss: detectability of technique, patient satisfaction, and classification. Plast Reconstr Surg 2008;122:13011311.
20. Hurwitz DJ. Boomerang pattern correction of gynecomastia. Plast Reconstr Surg 2015;135(2): 433–6.
21. Hurwitz DJ, Beidas O, Wright L. Reshaping the oversized waist through oblique flankplasty with lipoabdominoplasty (OFLA). Plast Reconstr Surg 2019;5: 960–72.
22. Webster J-P. Mastectomy for gynecomastia through semicircular intra-areolar incisions. Ann Surg 1946; 124:557.
23. Hurwitz DJ. In: Steinbrech D, editor. Chapter 22 boomerang excision pattern correction of gynecomastia in male aesthetic plastic surgery. New York: Thieme Publishers; 2021. p. 279–86.
24. Clavijo-Alvarez JA, Hurwitz DJ, Torsoplasty J. A novel approach to avoid circumferential scars of the upper body lift. Plast Reconstr Surg 2012; 130(2):382e–3e.
25. Villegas F. TULUA lipoabdominoplasty: no supraumbilical elevation combined with transverse infraumbilical plication, video description, and experience with 164 patients. Aesth Surg Journ 2021;41(5):594.
26. Hurwitz DJ. Body lift after massive weight loss in men. In: Steinbrech D, editor. Chapter 40 in aesthetic plastic surgery in men. New York: Thieme Publishers; 2021. p. 4987–5512.
27. Hurwitz D. Enhancing masculine features after massive weight loss. Aesth Plast Surg 2016;40(2): 245–55.

SUPPLEMENTARY DATA

Supplementary data to this article are found online at https://doi.org/10.1016/j.cps.2021.12.003.

REFERENCES

High-Definition Liposuction in Men

Michael J. Stein, MD, FRCSC[a,b,*], Alan Matarasso, MD, FACS[a,b]

KEYWORDS

- Male plastic surgery • Male aesthetics • Male liposuction • Male body contouring
- High-definition liposuction

KEY POINTS

- Liposuction has evolved from a procedure whose objective was primarily fat extraction to one which equally sculpts and redistributes fat in order to enhance natural muscular contours and shadows.
- Appropriate patient selection is necessary to perform HDL safely, effectively and reliably.
- Although numerous techniques can be used, the optimal technique is one tailored to the male's specific anatomy.

INTRODUCTION

Decades of innovation and technical refinement has made liposuction a safe, reliable, and reproducible procedure that is associated with high patient satisfaction.[1] Liposuction is the most common aesthetic procedure performed worldwide, and its popularity is increasing, with a 24% increase from 2014 to 2018.[2,3] In 2018, expenditures exceeded 1.3 billion dollars in the United States alone. Increasing obesity rates, improved visibility through social media, and an increasing number of patients seeking body contouring with minimal downtime has fueled its rapid increase in popularity and broadening indications for use.

Traditional liposuction, which is typically performed in the deep subcutaneous plane, was popularized as an effective way to extract fat and treat moderate to severe lipodystrophy of one or more body areas. Superficial liposuction, or debulking of the fat layer above the fascia superficialis (Scarpas, Colles, or Campers fascia based on its anatomical area), was historically approached with caution, as it was associated with an increase in complications such as induration, fibrosis, seroma, and contour irregularities.[4] A variety of technological adjuncts emerged over the years, such as ultrasound, laser, power, and radiofrequency-assisted liposuction devices, yet all predominantly targeted fat in the deep subcutaneous plane, and served to facilitate more efficient fat extraction and soft tissue contraction.

Recently, superficial liposuction has re-emerged as a finesse body contouring technique that enhances muscular definition. The idea that differential liposuction could be performed in the superficial plane around muscle groups to enhance aesthetic outcomes was initially described in the 1990s by Mentz,[5] Fodor,[6] and Ersek.[7] This technique, which the investigators referred to as "abdominal etching," exhibited superior aesthetics in contouring the male abdomen compared to traditional liposuction maneuvers. Specifically, the investigators demonstrated that stubborn subdermal fat was responsible for obscuring the final muscular contour following traditional techniques, and removing differential thicknesses of fat around these muscles illuminated them and enhanced their postoperative

Received: Jan 1, 2022.
[a] Manhattan Eye, Ear and Throat Hospital, 210 E 64th St, New York, NY 10065, USA; [b] Lenox Hill Hospital, 100 E 77th St, New York, NY 10075, USA
* Corresponding author.
E-mail address: mike.stein@nychhc.org

Clin Plastic Surg 49 (2022) 307–312
https://doi.org/10.1016/j.cps.2022.01.003

apperance. Although the described techniques were limited to contouring of the male abdomen, the concept that liposuction could now "sculpt" fat, instead of simply removing it, was born, and the demographic of patients presenting for liposuction slowly broadened.

Restricting patient selection to abdominal contouring in men with relatively low body mass indices, a steep technical learning curve, and persistent fear of complications tempered widespread adoption of these early techniques. In the late 2000s, however, Hoyos[8,9] described, and subsequently popularized, a modified, more comprehensive technique, that expanded on original principles to include 3-dimensional contouring of the entire body. "High-definition liposuction" (HDL), now applied to both sexes, at varying degrees of body fat percentages, and used vibration amplification of sound energy resonance (VASER) technology to facilitate enhanced sculpting. VASER-assisted HDL emphasized selective fat retention and removal in both superficial and deep layers to generate more natural and highly defined muscular units. The goal was fat sculpting rather than fat debulking. Fat was first prepared by emulsification, followed by the selective sculpting by gentle extraction aspiration around natural body convexities and concavities. Hoyos emphasized the importance of addressing "dynamic zones" of the body, where surgeons would anticipate the precise muscle movements during physical activity and sculpt the fat in a complementary fashion to avoid artificial-looking results. Increasing evidence over the coming years supporting HDL's safety, reliability, and aesthetic outcomes lead to its gradual adoption among the plastic surgery community.

Today, HDL has become common in the public vernacular. Improved visibility via social media has made the procedure increasingly popular, particularly among male patients. Patient perception has colloquially morphed liposuction into 2 separate procedures; the "traditional" or "basic" liposuction for fat extraction and the "new" or "advanced" high-definition technique. In the authors' practice, we find patients calling to specifically ask if the surgeon performs the "new type" of liposuction. Patients seem to be motivated to seek a surgeon who is equipped with the tools and experience to perform these techniques.

As enthusiasm for this procedure continues to grow, surgeons must equip themselves with the knowledge and techniques to appropriately select patients for the procedure, counsel them accordingly, and execute the procedure safely and effectively. Herein, we present important aspects of HDL anatomy, patient selection, surgical technique, and outcomes.

SUBCUTANEOUS FAT ANATOMY

Surgeons performing HDL must appreciate the regional differences in subcutaneous anatomy throughout the human body. The relative thickness of superficial and deep subcutaneous layers and the density of the fibroseptal network within these layers differ topographically across the body. As such, liposuction technique must be modified accordingly.

The superficial subcutaneous layer is characterized by dense fat lobules within an organized and compact strattice of fibroseptal fibers. The deeper layer, which is considerably thicker in areas of fat accumulation such as the abdomen and inner thighs, is characterized by larger and looser fat lobules, and a more haphazard fibroseptal network arrangement.[10]

Key zones of adherence throughout the body must also be recognized to prevent contour irregularities.[11] These include the lateral gluteal depression, gluteal crease, posterior thigh, inferolateral thigh overlying the iliotibial band, and the mid-medial thigh. These zones are characterized by a thin deep subcutaneous layer and dense fibroseptal network attachment tethering the superficial fascia to the deep muscular fascia. The paucity of deep subcutaneous fat in these areas lead to easy cannula misadventure into the superficial plane, increasing the risk for contour irregularities.

The fibroseptal network is also responsible for cellulite, a common presenting complaint of patients presenting for liposuction. While the pathophysiology of cellulite formation is not fully understood, the strutural orientation of the collagen septae, as well as hormonal and inflammatory etiologies have been proposed. While cellulite occurs in 80 to 98% of postpubertal women, it is uncommon in males, but can occur when males with androgen deficiency or who take estrogen therapy.[12] Two types of cellulite have been described. Type I cellulite, which is considered genetically predetermined, results from fat hypertrophy around fibroseptal network dermal tether points (classicly seen in the legs and buttocks). They are more commonly found in women, occur at a younger age, and are unrelated to the degree of adiposity or overall body shape. Type II cellulite, on the other hand, results from skin laxity and is more common in elderly patients with poor skin quality.[13]

Key intergender and interracial differences in fat distribution also exist. Men classically present with an android pattern of fat distribution, with an evenly distributed accumulation of fat centrally and a linear shape to the body. They tend to accumulate fat in the abdomen and superolateral hips. Women classically present with a gynoid fat distribution, which is most prominent in the gluteofemoral region posteriorly and inferiorly, resulting in a curvilinear body shape. These distributions must be preserved (and at times enhanced) during liposuction to attain aesthetic results and prevent inappropriate feminization or masculinization of the body. Interracial differences similarly exist. The distribution of body fat for women of the same BMI differs by race in reproductive-aged women, with some ethnic backgrounds accumulating more fat in the buttocks and hips than others.[14,15] It is important to respect these cultural preferences and cosmetic ideals when performing high-definition liposuction in men.

PATIENT SELECTION

Not all male patients are liposuction candidates, and HDL candidacy is even more selective. Appropriate patient selection and risk stratification is critical to performing the procedure safely and reliably. A thorough past medical and surgical history, and review of medications, supplements, allergies, and social and family histories are all critical in screening for risk factors. In our practice we consider nonobese patients with good skin quality and mild to moderate fat excess. They should have a BMI less than 30, maintain a healthy lifestyle, exercise regularly, have a stable weight for 12 months, and exemplify appropriate expectations. Ideally patients have no medical or psychiatric comorbidities, and if they have a history of smoking, they are asked to refrain for 4 weeks preoperatively. Any comorbidities warrant preoperative assessment and clearance from a primary care provider.

Poor candidates for HDL have unrealistic expectations, may exhibit features of body dysmorphia during the consultation, and have a history of massive weight loss or poor skin quality. Patients with skin excess will be disappointed with HDL alone. While select patients with mild skin excess and laxity can be treated effectively with radiofrequency-assisted devices during HDL, most cases require concomitant or delayed excisional procedures to attain the optimal aesthetic. Patients should be counseled accordingly.

We provide a list of medications and supplements to prospective patients that are associated with an increased risk for bleeding or clotting , or which may interfere with lidocaine metabolism. We require all patients to seize supplementation

and/or hormonal therapy for at least 4 weeks before surgery. If the patient takes nonsteroidal antiinflammatories, they are held for 2 weeks before surgery. We calculate a Caprini score for each patient to assess their risk of venous thromboembolic event (VTE) and anticoagulate patients and/or refer them to a hematologist as necessary.

SURGICAL TECHNIQUE

A "one-size-fits-all" approach to HDL must be avoided. Optimizing results requires the surgeon to tailor their technique to the specific body type and anatomy. Body biotype, metabolic state, patient age, race, sociocultural factors, and preoperative expectations all must be considered to prevent unnatural results.[16] Small volume HDL cases can be performed under local or general anesthesia based on patient health status and comfort level. HDL in the context of high-volume liposuction, concomitant procedures, or 2 or more areas are performed under general anesthesia. Cases are done in an ambulatory fashion with lipoaspirate volumes kept less than five liters.

Patient Preparation

Patients are dressed in a surgical gown and compression stockings, and standardized preoperative photographs are taken. The patient is then marked in the standing position, with black to indicate anatomic landmarks such as boney prominences, green to indicate areas of volume reduction where liposuction is primarily done in the deep plane, and red to demarcate inscriptions (ie, linea semilunaris, linea alba and transverse inscriptions) and zones of transition (also known as negative spaces or shadow areas), where liposuction is done more superficially. Blue crosshatches are placed in areas that will be augmented with fat grafting. In males, it is particularly important to ask them to contract muscle groups in different body positions to help illuminate "dynamic zones"[17]. Zones of transition are therefore not marked as distinct lines but a rectangle reflecting muscle position in resting versus contracted states.Without marking dynamic muscle contraction, liposculpting in males looks artificial and unnatural. After marking the patient, standardized photographs with markings are repeated in the same views.

Patients are prewarmed with a Bair Hugger and premedicated with antiemetic and nonsteroidal antiinflammatories. A lower body Bair Hugger is placed on the operating room bed, under a sterile blue drape. Sequential compression devices are placed upon entering the room. A surgical pause is performed, at the end of which we review and post on the operating room monitor the patient's weight, maximal allowed volume of tumescent solution using a maximum limit of 35 mg/kg, and the planned volume of infiltration (total and per area). A cephalosporin antibiotic is administered at the start of the case and redosed as necessary.

Surgical Technique

The least number of incisions to facilitate maximal access to the treated area is chosen. Having said this, men commonly require more incisions than women to gain access to inscriptions, and surgeons should not compromise the surgical result by limiting access points. Where possible, incisions are strategically placed in skin creases or along undergarment lines. If incisions cannot be hidden, such as in the central back in men, we purposefully place incisions asymmetrically. Tumescent infiltration is performed with a roller pump through an exploded tip cannula MicroAire handpiece (Surgical Instruments, Charlottesville, VA), using the simultaneous separation and tumescence technique (SST). A solution of 1000 mL Ringers Lactate, 1mL of 1:1000 epinephrine, 50 mL of 1% lidocaine (500mg) and 10 mL of 8.4% sodium bicarbonate is used. Although it has been shown that the optimal waiting time until maximal hemostatic effect is 26 minutes,[18] we typically wait 10 minutes before proceeding with aspiration. Fat emulsification using the VASER probe has been championed by investigators such as Hoyos and allows for smooth and effective fat extraction. In our practice, aesthetic results can be achieved with power-assisted liposuction (PAL) alone, which we find decreases operative time, surgical costs, and risk of skin burns. VASER is preferentially used for secondary liposuction cases in which there is more tissue fibrosis. Aspiration is performed in the deep plane with a Mercedes cannula, the size of which depends on the body area (4–5 mm for trunk, 3–4 mm for extremities). Next, controlled deformities are created over inscriptions in the superficial plane with an exploded tip cannula. This is tapered laterally in order to accentuate zones of transition. Unlike in women, who are best treated with gradual tapering, the male aesthetic requires sharper and more obvious transition zone around muscle groups. The nondominant hand guides the cannula trajectory, and pinch tests are used to assess thickness and symmetry between sides.

In cases where fat grafting augmentation is added to the procedure, we prepare the fat by decantation and transfer them into syringes for manual injection. All fat grafting is performed in the subcutaneous and not the intramuscular plane, irrespective of anatomic area. The pectoralis and deltoid muscles, so-called male "alpha" muscles, require volume to further exentuate the transition zone created with HDL. The rectus muscles on the other hand, seldom requires fat grafting as HDL alone will accentuate contour sufficiently. If performed, modest volumes are injected, as the recti quickly adopt an artificial static apperance, discordant with their dynamic contraction. Following fat grafting, all incisions are closed with a deep dermal monocryl sutures followed by nylon simple interrupted sutures. Drains are only used in high-volume liposuction cases.

Postoperative Care

Foam cut outs are placed over inscriptions and areas of superficial liposculpting, and a compression garment is placed over top. This garment is worn continuously for 48 hours and then taken off for the first shower. The patient is encouraged to shower daily and begin lymphatic massages at this point. For 2 weeks the patient is encouraged to use the foam cut outs and surgical compression garment. After 2 weeks they can remove the foam and wear the compression garment of their choosing. It is worth noting that the patient must try on their own compression garment at a follow-up visit so it can be assessed by their surgeon. Inappropriately fitted garments can lead to hyperpigmentation, skin irritation, and even full-thickness skin necrosis.

Select patients who undergo concomitant procedures or high-volume liposuction are monitored overnight. Otherwise, patients are discharged with a chaperone and encouraged to ambulate immediately and regularly. All patients are discharged with an information packet about their postoperative course, a list of red flags to look out for, and contact information should they have any concerns postoperatively.

High-Definition Liposuction as Concomitant Procedure

HDL is increasingly being used concomitantly with excisional procedures, such as abdominoplasty,[19,20] gynecomastia surgery,[17,21] brachioplasty,[22] and fat grafting.[23–25] Although it can be performed before or after skin excision, our practice is to perform it first, as it helps facilitate maximal skin resection. If HDL is performed first, the surgeon must mimic the vector of skin redraping following excision and mark inscriptions and transition zones accordingly. For instance, during the male abdominoplasty, the skin flap is cheated medially upon closure to avoid "dog ear" formation. If rectus diastasis is performed, the rectus abdominis muscles will also be medialized. If HDL is performed without consideration of these post-resection changes, sculpted inscriptions and transition zones will be inappropriately positioned. Preoperative markings must mimic anticipated vectors of skin advancement and the HDL performed accordingly. In the author's practice we have adopted HDL as a routine adjunct to male abdominoplasties, brachioplasties and gynecomatstia surgeries.

OUTCOMES

The most common complications following HDL are seroma and contour irregularities. Bruising, and rarely, hematoma are possible. Rare major complication of liposuction in general includes VTE, fat embolism, skin necrosis, lidocaine toxicity, and visceral perforation.[26,27]

Outcomes following HDL have been recently described in multiple retrospective reviews. Saad's retrospective case series of 50 men undergoing HDL categorized cases into high definition, moderate definition, and mild definition. The high-definition group had the highest patient satisfaction but the highest incidence of minor complications (21%).[28] High patient satisfaction with minimal morbidity was also noted in reviews of HDL cases by Nidaam[29] and Saad.[30,31] Danilla reviewed 417 patients who underwent HDL, 333 (80%) of whom were men, and 29% of those who underwent concomitant procedures. Most patients (94%) were happy with their results, there were no major complications, and minor complications included hyperpigmentation, seroma, nodular fibrosis, unsatisfactory definition, unnatural appearance, and VASER-related burns.[32] A large series by Agochukwu-Nwubah of 512 male HDL cases noted the only complication being contour defects in only 3 patients, with no infections, skin necrosis, or seroma.[33] Recently, a systematic review by Escandon reviewed data from 13 studies and 1280 male patients undergoing HDL. Most studies used power-assisted liposuction alone (6 studies) followed by conventional liposuction (4 studies) and VASER-assisted liposuction (3 studies). Overall satisfaction was high (84%–100%), and the most common complications were seroma, hyperpigmentation, contour irregularities, anemia, and port dehiscence.[34]

SUMMARY

The market for male aesthetic surgery has increased exponentially over the last two decades. Male liposuction candidates historically included those with moderate to severe lipodystrophy seeking a weight loss procedure. Now the demographic has morphed into one dominated by young, athletic men with mild to moderate lipodystrophy and high expectations for a sculpted and enhanced muscular apperance. A review of the literature supports a safe, reliable, and reproducible procedure in the appropriately selected patient. Surgeons can achieve favorable results with appropriate patient selection, preoperative counseling on realistic expectations, and adherence to the technical principles described in the literature.

CLINICS CARE POINTS

- High-Definition Liposuction (HDL) is not suitable for all male patients. Careful patient selection is a critical prerequisite to ensure safe and reliable results.

- Surgeons must appreciate the unique anatomical characteristics of the fat, fibroseptal network and muscle groups in the area being treated. Liposuction of transition zones, dynamic contraction zones and unique muscular inscription arrangements is necessary to create a natural-appearing result.

- When HDL is performed concomitantly with excisional procedures, it is performed before skin resection. In order to ensure appropriately placed muscular inscriptions and transition zones following HDL, the preoperative markings must anticipate skin mobilization following closure.

DISCLOSURE

Dr M.J. Stein and Dr A. Matarasso have no disclosure.[13]

REFERENCES

1. Mendez BM, Coleman JE, Kenkel JM. Optimizing patient outcomes and safety with liposuction. Aesthet Surg J 2019;39(1):66–82.
2. Cosmetic surgery national data bank statistics. Aesthet Surgy J 2017;37(suppl2):1–29.
3. American Society of Plastic Surgeons. Plastic surgery statistics report 2019: ASPS national clearinghouse of plastic surgery procedural statistics 2019. Available at: https://www.plasticsurgery.org/documents/News/Statistics/2019/plastic-surgerystatistics-full-report-2019.pdf. Accessed December 20, 2021.
4. Avelar J. Regional distribution and behavior of the subcutaneous tissue concerning selection and indication for liposuction. Aesthetic Plast Surg 1989; 13(3):155–65.

5. Mentz HA 3rd, Gilliland MD, Patronella CK. Abdominal etching: differential liposuction to detail abdominal musculature. Aesthet Plast Surg 1993;17(4):287–90.

6. Fodor PB. Superficial liposuction. Aesthet Surg J 1993;13:10–4.

7. Ersek RA, Salisbury AV. Abdominal etching. Aesthetic Plast Surg 1997;21:328–31.

8. Hoyos AE. High definition liposculpture. Presented in the XIII International Course of Plastic Surgery. Bucaramanga, Colombia, October 9, 2003.

9. Hoyos AE, Millard JA. VASER-assisted high-definition liposculpture. Aesthet Surg J 2007;27(6):594–604.

10. Markman B, Barton FE Jr. Anatomy of the subcutaneous tissue of the trunk and lower extremity. Plast Reconstr Surg 1987;80(2):248–54.

11. Rohrich RJ, Smith PD, Marcantonio DR, et al. The zones of adherence: role in minimizing and preventing contour deformities in liposuction. Plast Reconstr Surg 2001;107(6):1562–9.

12. Avram MM. Cellulite: a review of its physiology and treatment. J Cosmet Laser Ther 2005;6:181-5.

13. Mendez BM. Mendez BM, Coleman JE, Kenkel JM. Optimizing Patient Outcomes and Safety With Liposuction. Aesthet Surg J. 2019 Jan 1;39(1):66-82. Aesthet Surg J. 2019. https://doi.org/10.1093/asj/sjy151.

14. Kanaley JA, Giannopoulou I, Tillapaugh-Fay G, et al. Racial differences in subcutaneous and visceral fat distribution in postmenopausal black and white women. Metabolism 2003;52(2):186–91.

15. Rahman M, Temple JR, Breitkopf CR, et al. Racial differences in body fat distribution among reproductive-aged women. Metabolism 2009;58(9):1329–37.

16. Hoyos AE, Perez ME, Domínguez-Millán R. Variable sculpting in dynamic definition body contouring: procedure selection and management algorithm. Aesthet Surg J 2021;41(3):318–32.

17. Hoyos A, Perez M. Dynamic-definition male pectoral reshaping and enhancement in slim, athletic, obese, and gynecomastic patients through selective fat removal and grafting. Aesthet Plast Surg 2012;36(5):1066–77.

18. McKee DE, Lalonde DH, Thoma A, et al. Optimal time delay between epinephrine injection and incision to minimize bleeding. Plast Reconstr Surg 2013;131(4):811–4.

19. Hoyos A, Perez ME, Guarin DE, et al. A report of 736 high-definition lipoabdominoplasties performed in conjunction with circumferential VASER liposuction. Plast Reconstr Surg 2018;142(3):662–75.

20. Simão TS. High definition lipoabdominoplasty. Aesthet Plast Surg 2020;44(6):2147–57.

21. Hoyos AE, Perez ME, Domínguez-Millán R. Gynecomastia treatment through open resection and pectoral high-definition liposculpture. Plast Reconstr Surg 2021;147(5):1072–83.

22. Hoyos A, Perez M. Arm dynamic definition by liposculpture and fat grafting. Aesthet Surg J 2012;32(8):974–87.

23. Steinbrech DS, Sinno S. Utilizing the power of fat grafting to obtain a naturally-appearing muscular "6-pack" abdomen. Aesthet Surg J 2016;36:1085–8.

24. Hoyos AE, Perez ME, Domínguez-Millán R. Male aesthetics for the gluteal area: anatomy and algorithm for surgical approach for dynamic definition body contouring. Plast Reconstr Surg 2020;146(2):284–93.

25. Danilla S. Rectus abdominis fat transfer (RAFT) in lipoabdominoplasty: a new technique to achieve fitness body contour in patients that require tummy tuck. Aesthet Plast Surg 2017;41(6):1389–99.

26. Lehnhardt M, Homann HH, Daigeler A, et al. Major and lethal complications of liposuction: a review of 72 cases in Germany between 1998 and 2002. Plast Reconstr Surg 2008;121(6):396e–403e.

27. Kaoutzanis C, Gupta V, Winocour J, et al. Cosmetic liposuction: preoperative risk factors, major complication rates, and safety of combined procedures. Aesthet Surg J 2017;37(6):680–94.

28. Saad A, Altamirano-Arcos CA, Nahas Combina L, et al. Power-assisted liposculpture in male patients: a spectrum of definitions. Aesthet Surg J 2021;41(6):NP447–55.

29. Niddam J, Hersant B, Aboud C, et al. Postoperative complications and patient satisfaction after abdominal etching: prospective case series of 25 patients. Aesthet Plast Surg 2020;44(3):830–5.

30. Saad AN, Arbelaez JP, de Benito J. High definition liposculpture in male patients using reciprocating power-assisted liposuction technology: techniques and results in a prospective study. Aesthet Surg J 2019;40(3):299–307.

31. Saad A, Combina LN, Altamirano-Arcos C. Abdominal etching. Clin Plast Surg 2020;47(3):397–408.

32. Danilla S, Babaitis RA, Jara RP, et al. High-definition liposculpture: what are the complications and how to manage them? Aesthet Plast Surg 2020;44(2):411–8.

33. Agochukwu-Nwubah N, Mentz HA. Abdominal etching: past and present. Aesthet Surg J 2019;39(12):1368–77.

34. Escandón JM, Vyas KS, Manrique OJ. High-definition lipoplasty in male patients: a systematic review of surgical techniques and outcomes. Aesthet Surg J 2022;42(1):68–85.

Calf Augmentation

Paul N. Chugay, MD

KEYWORDS

- Calf hypoplasia • Club foot • Shapely leg

KEY POINTS

- Implant selection is paramount, making sure that the right implant is chosen to meet the patient's needs without exceeding the capacity of the leg based on preoperative measurements and the surgeon's assessment of esthetics.
- Careful and judicious dissection is key to this procedure. Overdissection results in extra dead space that can result in seroma, hematoma, and possible implant malposition.
- Avoidance of injury to the short saphenous vein that runs in the midline posteriorly and lays deep to the investing fascia of the leg along the surface of the gastrocnemius.
- Layered closure with absorbable sutures ensures a more esthetically pleasing scar postoperatively.
- Wrap for compression in the first 24 hours to minimize implant mobility and keep swelling compartmentalized. Postoperative use of compression stockings with a grading of 20 to 30 mm Hg helps to minimize the dead space and the risk of implant movement until scar tissue has developed.

INTRODUCTION

A well-sculpted calf is something often sought after by male patients presenting for cosmetic surgery. Despite hours in the gym doing calf raises, lunges, and squats, some men are not able to achieve the volume and definition desired in the calf region. Using semisolid silicone prostheses, a man with thin legs can achieve a more athletic masculine contour. Via a 5 cm incision in the popliteal fossa, implants can be placed to augment the medial head of the gastrocnemius, the lateral head of the gastrocnemius, or provide overall volume augmentation of the calf to produce a more bulky calf region. Regardless of the implants used, calf augmentation is a straightforward and reproducible procedure that provides excellent results in the vast majority of male patients presenting for improvement in perceived disproportion of the leg.

HISTORY OF THE PROCEDURE

Over the course of the last 40 years since the introduction of calf augmentation for reconstructive purposes, there have been various surgeons who have proposed novel implant shapes and sizes along with varying locations for the placement of the implants.[1–12] The implant most commonly used today is largely based on the silicone gel implants of Glitzenstein. However, Carlsen was the first to use calf implants back in 1972.[13] His initial implant was made out of silastic foam. Glitzenstein, in 1979, used calf implants for patients with atrophy of the leg and muscular aplasia. Unlike Carlsen, his implants were designed from silicone gel. In 1984, Szalay introduced torpedo-shaped implants that were placed beneath the fascia. In his technique, however, he did recommend the use of relaxing incisions in the fascia.[4] Aiache in 1991 introduced lenticular-shaped implants.[12] In 2006, Gutstein described a new silicone prosthesis that enhances the curved medial lower leg, which he termed a "combined calf-tibial implant."[7]

The early pioneers of the procedure, Carlsen and Glizenstein, introduced the implant into a subfascial plane. However, in 2003, Kalixto and Vergara[6] described a calf augmentation with placement of the implant in a submuscular pocket, between the gastrocnemius and soleus muscles. The dissection that they proposed was done far away from the union of the gastrocnemius muscles where there were no vessels or nerves that could

Private Practice - Chugay Cosmetic Surgery, 4210 Atlantic Avenue, Long Beach, CA 90807, USA
E-mail address: Docchugay@hotmail.com

Clin Plastic Surg 49 (2022) 313–328
https://doi.org/10.1016/j.cps.2021.12.007
0094-1298/22/© 2022 Elsevier Inc. All rights reserved.

be damaged. It was noted, however, that these patients had a more tedious dissection and prolonged recovery than the patients who had undergone subfascial implant placement as described in previous reports. Use of muscle relaxants was paramount in these patients. The rationale for submuscular placement, according to the authors, was that they were able to gain better camouflaging of the implant. In 2004, Nunes described a method for calf augmentation that placed the implant in a supraperiosteal plane associated with fasciotomies. Ultimately, it is at the surgeon's discretion where to place the implant; however, based on anatomic studies, it seems that the subfascial plane is a safe plane that allows for reproducible results with minimal risk of postoperative complications and significantly less pain from the patient's perspective.[11] It is for this reason that the author favors a subfascial plane in the medial aspect of the calf for the vast majority of augmentations.

RELEVANT ANATOMY

As a result of anatomic studies[11] and operative dissections, the anatomy of the calf region is well understood. The calf is made up of 2 muscle groups: the gastrocnemius and the soleus (**Fig. 1**). The gastrocnemius has 2 heads and lies superficial to the deeper soleus muscle.

The fibers of the 2 heads unite at an angle in the midline of the muscle in a tendinous raphe, which expands into a broad aponeurosis. The aponeurosis, gradually contracting, unites with the tendon of the soleus and forms the calcaneal tendon (Achilles tendon). In performing the dissection to attain a subfascial plane, the lateral and medial cutaneous nerves, branches of the peroneal nerve and tibial nerve, respectively, are potentially

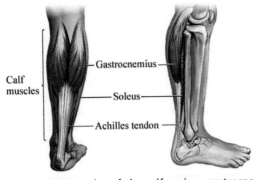

Fig. 1. Major muscles of the calf region: gastrocnemius and soleus. (*From* Chugay PN. Chapter 35: Calf Augmentation. In: Steinbrech, DS, ed. Male Aesthetic Plastic Surgery. 1st ed. Thieme; 2020:420.)

encountered. These nerves provide sensory innervation to the skin (**Fig. 2**). The medial sural cutaneous nerve originates from the tibial nerve of the sciatic and descends between the 2 heads of the gastrocnemius. It can be identified before diving between the heads of the gastrocnemius in the upper midline calf region. The lateral sural cutaneous nerve supplies the skin on the posterior and lateral surfaces of the leg and travels in a subcutaneous plane alongside the small (short) saphenous vein, joining with the medial sural cutaneous nerve to form the sural nerve. Major arterial, venous, and nerve structures are deep within the calf and remain undisturbed during a routine calf augmentation procedure (**Fig. 3**). The subfascial plane, both medially and laterally, is relatively avascular, allowing for the creation of a relatively bloodless plane. That being said, care must be taken to avoid injury to the short saphenous vein which lay deep to the investing fascia of the leg and superficial to the gastrocnemius in the midline posteriorly. This vein drains into the popliteal vein in the popliteal fossa. Care must be exercised when placing implants to produce a more "bulky" calf as this implant spans the midline and injury to the short saphenous vein is a risk.

INDICATIONS

Calf augmentation was originally designed to fill defects left following oncologic surgery, after trauma or infection, or due to genetic abnormalities that left patients with a "shrunken" lower leg. There are many causes for unilateral or bilateral calf deformities and they include but are not limited to the following: (1) congenital hypoplasia due to agenesis of a calf muscle or adipose tissue reduction; (2) as sequelae of clubfoot (talipes equinovarus), cerebral palsy, polio, and spina bifida; (3) due to poliomyelitis or osteomyelitis; and (4) following fractures of the femur and as a result of burn contractures.[1,2,13,14] Since its initial introduction, calf augmentation surgery has become a widely popular esthetic procedure to help patients gain more shapely legs. Bodybuilders and some male sports enthusiasts may want to demonstrate a more bulky leg or what we like to term the "football calf." Other men, presenting for surgery, may just want to have some increased volume in the medial and/or lateral calf to produce a more gentle curve and shapely leg. Ultimately, it is a simple disproportion between the thigh and calf that brings patients in for surgery. Using silicone implants, one can bring about greater harmony to the male leg and produce a more muscular and "masculine" leg.

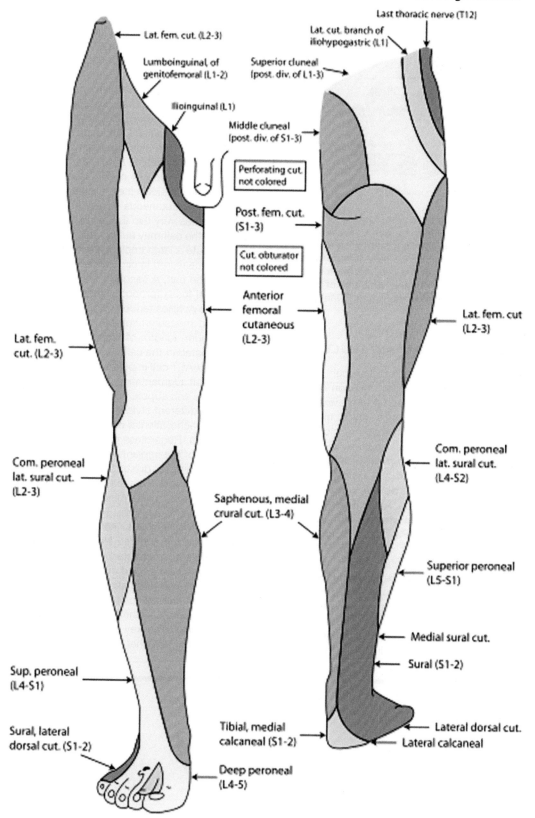

Last thoracic nerve (T12)

Lat. cut. branch of
iliohypogastric (L1)

Lat. fem. cut. (L2-3)

Lumboinguinal of
genitofemoral (L1-2)

Superior cluneal
(post. div. of L1-3)

Ilioinguinal (L1)

Middle cluneal
(post. div. of S1-3)

Perforating cut.
not colored

Post. fem. cut.
(S1-3)

Cut. obturator
not colored

Anterior
femoral
cutaneous
(L2-3)

Lat. fem. cut
(L2-3)

Lat. fem.
cut. (L2-3)

Com. peroneal
lat. sural cut.
(L4-S2)

Com. peroneal
lat. sural cut.
(L2-3)

Saphenous, medial
crural cut. (L3-4)

Superior peroneal
(L5-S1)

Medial sural cut.

Sural (S1-2)

Sup. peroneal
(L4-S1)

Sural, lateral
dorsal cut. (S1-2)

Tibial, medial
calcaneal (S1-2)

Lateral dorsal cut.

Lateral calcaneal

Deep peroneal
(L4-5)

Fig. 2. The lateral and medial cutaneous nerves dermatomes are seen here. These are branches of the peroneal nerve and tibial nerve, respectively, and are potentially encountered in dissection for calf augmentation. These nerves provide sensory innervation to the skin in the area. (*Adapted from* Gray H. Anatomy of the Human Body. https://www.bartleby.com/107/indexillus.html.)

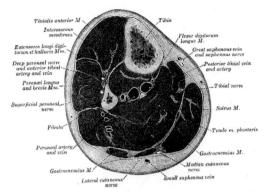

Fig. 3. Major neurovascular structures are seen in this cross-section of the midportion of the calf. When performing a subfascial augmentation (as is our standard), these structures are relatively safe from injury as most major structures are deep to the muscle of the calf. (*Adapted from* Gray H. Anatomy of the Human Body. https://www.bartleby.com/107/indexillus.html.)

THE CONSULTATION/IMPLANT SELECTION

The consultation begins with a thorough medical history of the patient. Special attention is taken to ask specifically about trauma to the extremity, history of surgery to the foot or ankle, history of vascular insufficiency which may put blood flow at risk, history of venous insufficiency or leg swelling which may prolong postoperative edema in the lower extremity, and any history of nerve damage or sensory deficits as may be seen in patients with diabetes mellitus. At the time of consultation, the patient is asked what specifically about their calf bothers them. Patients with unrealistic goals are deemed poor candidates for calf augmentation. Patients who have congenital anomalies, a significant size disparity between the 2 calves, or bilateral hypoplasia are informed that several surgeries may be required to attain symmetry and achieve the augmentation they desire. In the typical consultation, patients are asked if their deficiency lies primarily in the medial

aspect of the calf, the lateral aspect of the calf, or whether they would like a larger calf size overall. The reason for this distinction is to help the surgeon select the right implant style for the surgery.

After completion of the history, the patient's calves are evaluated. First, symmetry of the 2 sides is assessed and any disparity is brought to the attention of the patient. Although most patients present with a pre-existing asymmetry of the calves, not many patients note the difference and this can be a source of medicolegal matters in the future. The physician then evaluates the quality of the skin, subcutaneous tissue, and muscle. A person who has very thin tissues or significant hypoplasia of the calf may not be able to adequately accommodate a large implant. Next, the patient's calves are measured in circumference at the midportion of the calf. A second measurement, from the popliteal fossa (proposed incision line) to the origin of the Achilles tendon, is also taken. Having this second measurement allows one to assess the maximum length of implant that can be accommodated in the calf.

We favor AART calf implants (**Fig. 4**) as they provide sufficient augmentation of the region while still being pliable and supple, more like natural tissue. Each of the different style implants has a range of sizes to fit each patient's need (http://aartinc.net/calf-implants). Regardless of the implant chosen, the position of the implant is still in the subfascial plane and minimizes dissection around key neurovascular structures. With experience, the surgeon will be better able to determine the best implant for each patient.

In reconstructive cases, the size of the defect is assessed and the affected leg is compared with the contralateral, unaffected leg. Using measurements as noted earlier and the surgeon's personal experience, the surgeon should be able to determine the best implant to suit the patient's needs. The goal in purely esthetic cases is to enlarge the calf volume. The key in both instances is to choose the implant that is right for the patient

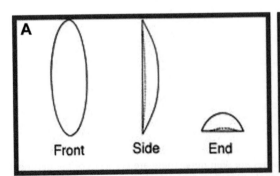

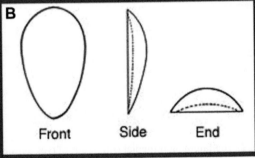

Fig. 4. (*A*) Calf implant style 2. (*B*) Calf implant style 1. (*Courtesy of* AART, Reno, NV.)

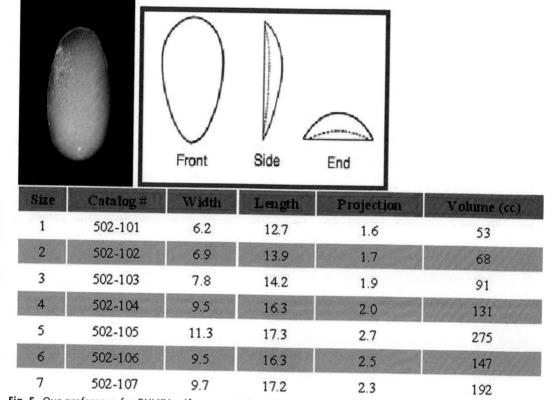

Size	Catalog #	Width	Length	Projection	Volume (cc)
1	502-101	6.2	12.7	1.6	53
2	502-102	6.9	13.9	1.7	68
3	502-103	7.8	14.2	1.9	91
4	502-104	9.5	16.3	2.0	131
5	502-105	11.3	17.3	2.7	275
6	502-106	9.5	16.3	2.5	147
7	502-107	9.7	17.2	2.3	192

Fig. 5. Our preference for BULKY calf augmentation. (*Courtesy of* AART, Reno, NV.)

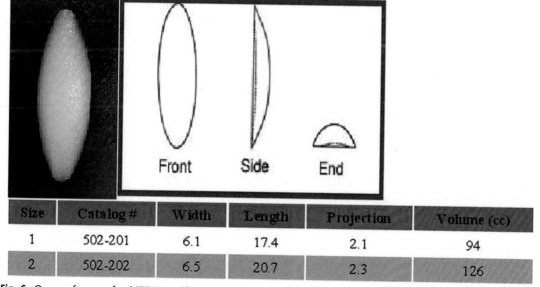

Size	Catalog #	Width	Length	Projection	Volume (cc)
1	502-201	6.1	17.4	2.1	94
2	502-202	6.5	20.7	2.3	126

Fig. 6. Our preference for MEDIAL calf augmentation. (*Courtesy of* AART, Reno, NV.)

rather than succumbing to the patient's demands. An implant that is too large may risk significant complications and may produce an unesthetic appearance.

Available Implants

Figs. 5–7.

PREOPERATIVE PLANNING AND MARKING

With the patient in the erect position, the proposed site of incision is marked, measuring approximately 5 cm. The site of incision should be in line with the patient's natural crease in the popliteal fossa. The exact popliteal crease can be accentuated by asking the patient to stand upright and hold on to a stationary object while flexing one knee at a time. Once the site of the incision is marked, the site of the proposed implant is marked taking into account the patient's anatomy and existing deficit along with the desires of the patient (**Fig. 8**).

OPERATIVE TECHNIQUE

The surgery is typically performed under general anesthesia or sedation to minimize patient discomfort. Two grams of Ancef are administered before the incision for prophylaxis (if allergic to penicillin or cephalosporin, then clindamycin 300 mg IV is administered). The patient is

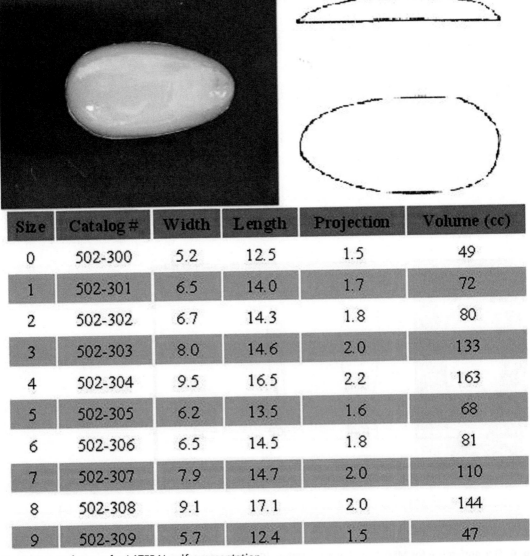

Size	Catalog #	Width	Length	Projection	Volume (cc)
0	502-300	5.2	12.5	1.5	49
1	502-301	6.5	14.0	1.7	72
2	502-302	6.7	14.3	1.8	80
3	502-303	8.0	14.6	2.0	133
4	502-304	9.5	16.5	2.2	163
5	502-305	6.2	13.5	1.6	68
6	502-306	6.5	14.5	1.8	81
7	502-307	7.9	14.7	2.0	110
8	502-308	9.1	17.1	2.0	144
9	502-309	5.7	12.4	1.5	47

Fig. 7. Our preference for LATERAL calf augmentation.

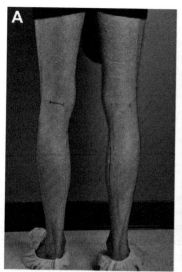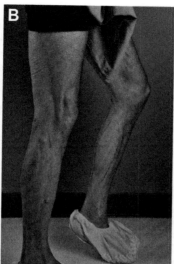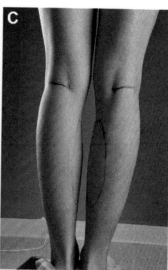

Fig. 8. (*A–C*) Preoperative markings for calf augmentation surgery. Note the site of the incision in the popliteal fossa and the outline of the site for calf augmentation. The markings for implant position are done in concert with the patient to maximize patient satisfaction postoperatively. Notice that the implants are placed in different positions in 5a and 5c, depending on the individual desires of the patient. NOTE: Anterior placement is limited by the investing fascia.

repositioned in the prone position after administration of anesthesia. The calves are then prepped with chlorhexidine and each calf is injected with a total of 50 cc of 1% lidocaine with epinephrine in the area of proposed implant placement. The patient is then reprepped and draped in a sterile fashion. A 5 cm incision is made in the popliteal fossa in line with preoperative markings. Subsequently, dissection is performed through the subcutaneous tissues. Dissection is carried to the level of the popliteal fascia. On reaching the fascia, a 15-blade scalpel is used to make a transverse incision (**Fig. 9**). This is extended with Metzenbaum scissors medially and laterally. At this point, 2-0 Vicryl stay sutures are placed in each section

of the fascia (**Fig. 10**). While performing this dissection, care is taken to avoid injury to the short saphenous vein which runs *in the midline* posteriorly and lays deep to the investing fascia of the leg along the surface of the gastrocnemius (**Fig. 11**). A subfascial plane, beginning beneath the popliteal fascia and extending into the deep investing fascia of the leg, is then dissected using blunt finger dissection and a spatula dissector, ensuring an adequate plane for the implant (in line with preoperative markings/patient wishes) (**Fig. 12**). Once a sufficient pocket is dissected, the pocket is irrigated with a solution containing normal saline, betadine, Ancef, and gentamicin. 15 cc of 0.5% Marcaine is injected into the pocket

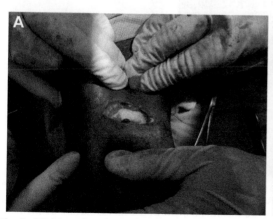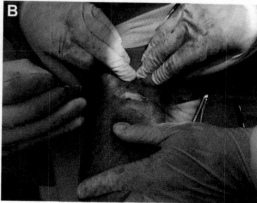

Fig. 9. (*A*) Dissection through the popliteal incision has been completed with blunt dissection and electrocautery to the level of the fascia. (*B*) With the fascia exposed, an incision in the fascia is made with a 15 blade producing a bulging of the subfascial fat. Metzenbaum scissors are used to widen the opening in the fascia.

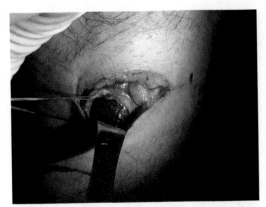

Fig. 10. The dissection of the gastrocnemius is complete. Stay sutures are placed into the cut edges of the fascia cephalically and caudally. The medial head of the gastrocnemius is fully exposed. The proposed site of implant is noted on the medial aspect of the leg (in red). NOTE: Notice the tissues laterally intact. Overaggressive dissection to the midline of the leg and laterally may damage the short saphenous vein.

skin is closed in a subcuticular fashion with 3-0 Monoderm Quill suture. The same procedure is mirrored on the contralateral side. An occlusive dressing is applied. The legs are wrapped with Coban, and the patient is then taken to the postanesthesia care unit (**Figs. 14–16**).

POSTOPERATIVE CARE/INSTRUCTIONS

Postoperatively the patient may begin ambulating starting on the evening of the procedure. They may shower POD 2, making sure to keep dressings clean and dry. Patients are then allowed to begin light activity at week 2 and full unrestricted activity at weeks 4 to 6. Patients are asked to wear compression stockings with a grading of 20 to 30 mm Hg for 4 weeks postoperatively to prevent dead space, thereby helping to reduce the risk of seroma formation and allowing scar tissue to form around the implant in the desired position. The legs are to be elevated as much as possible to allow for better lymphatic/venous drainage.

DISCUSSION

Although calf augmentation is a relatively straightforward procedure, there are complications that the surgeon should be aware of and that should be fully discussed with the patient preoperatively (**Box 1**).

for postoperative analgesia. An implant is then placed. Symmetry is assessed. At this point, closure is begun. The fascia is reapproximated with 2-0 Vicryl suture in an interrupted fashion (**Fig. 13**). The deep dermis is reapproximated with 3-0 Monocryl suture in a buried fashion. The

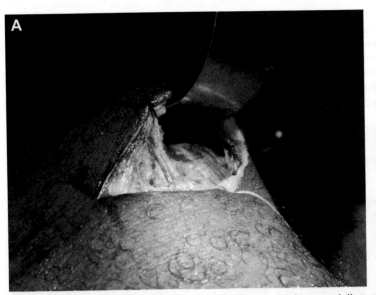
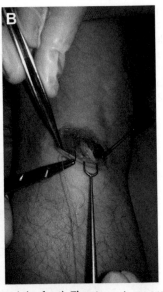

Fig. 11. (*A*) Dissection of the subfascial plane is complete (looking caudally toward the foot). The stay sutures are in place with the medial head of the gastrocnemius visible. The pocket has been dissected medially showing ample space for placement of the implant. Tissue planes are maintained, which allows for closure at the end. (*B*) Again, tissues in the midline of the calf are not violated for risk of damage to the short saphenous vein seen here depicted in the middle of the photo (bluish tinge at the point of the needle within the driver)—view is again looking caudally to the feet with the dissection for medial calf augmentation.

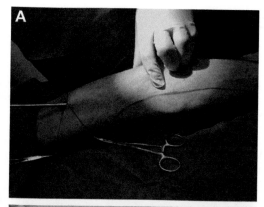

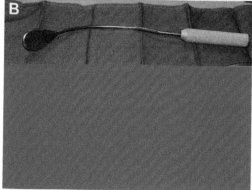

Fig. 12. (*A*) Dissection of the subfascial pocket using a spatula dissector, taking care to stay within the borders of the outlined implant. (*B*) A common spatula dissector frequently used in breast augmentation surgery that is quite useful in calf augmentation procedures.

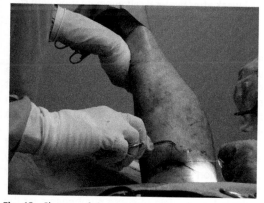

Fig. 13. Closure of the deep investing fascia of the leg using 2-0 Vicryl suture. To facilitate closure and take tension off of the ends of the fascia, the knee is flexed by the assistant.

Although the risk of infection is relatively low, ranging from 0[5] to 3.3%,[1] it can largely be avoided with good sterile surgical technique. Species identified in the author's experiences were isolated to *Staphylococcus aureus* and *Streptococcus epidermidis*, relatively common skin flora.

Seromas are statistically the most common complication occurring in calf augmentation surgery, occurring in approximately 6% of cases in most large volume studies.[4,11,15,16] The treatment of choice remains percutaneous aspiration. This complication is best prevented with patient compliance with compression stockings and avoidance of vigorous activity in the early post operative period and proper implant placement at the time of surgery, thereby minimizing dead space.

Although a rare occurrence, because of the relatively avascular plane of dissection for the calf augmentation procedure, a hematoma is always possible if damage is done to the vessels that perforate the investing fascia of the leg.[11] In the event of a hematoma, rapid evacuation, pocket irrigation, and reimplantation are the mainstays of therapy. This complication is best prevented by meticulous hemostasis at the time of surgery and good compression of the calf postoperative to prevent potential space creation.

Patients complaining of asymmetry and implant visibility are 2 complications that can be avoided by good preoperative consultation and evaluation. The vast majority of patients have a pre-existing asymmetry. This needs to be fully shown and discussed with the patient to avoid problems postoperatively. To avoid creating asymmetry with respect to implant position, the markings of the proposed site of implant placement should be thoroughly discussed and confirmed with the patient preoperatively. In cases of pre-existing asymmetry, creating greater asymmetry can be minimized by using a static anatomic structure such as the malleolus as a reference point for the implant tracings. With respect to implant visibility, all patients need to be made aware of thinner tissues that may be covering the implant may be more prone to revealing the borders of the implant versus a patient that has more subcutaneous tissue that can camouflage the implants.

Owing to the significant mobility in the calf region, hyperpigmented scars and hypertrophic scars along with wound dehiscence are indeed risks. To minimize these complications, the surgeon should be meticulous in his or her closure of the wound. By closing in anatomic layers and minimizing tension at the skin level, these risks may be lessened. To help in closure of the fascia, the patient's knee is flexed at the time of closure to

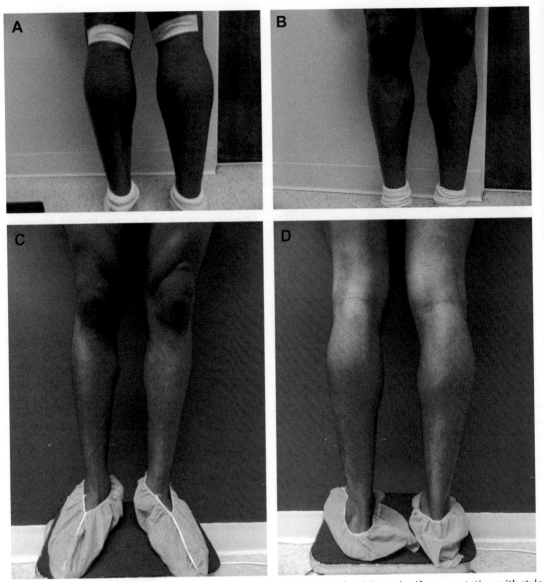

Fig. 14. Case 1: (*A–D*) A 42-year-old man is shown before and 1 week after bilateral calf augmentation with style 2, size 2 implants.

ensure good purchase of the fascia with the suture. Lastly, patients are asked to avoid overzealous activity for the first 4 to 6 weeks to again minimize tension on the scar. Without question, the use of scar gels and sunscreens can help to avoid a noticeable postoperative scar.

One of the possible late complications of calf augmentation is capsular contracture. The literature in calf augmentation has described a rate between 0%[3–5,10] and 5%.[1] If a patient presents with signs/symptoms of capsular contracture (eg, induration of the implant site, tightness in the leg, new-onset pain, new-onset swelling), ultrasound or CT evaluation of the affected extremity is warranted. If

a thickened capsule is identified, typically characterized by calcifications, then a partial or complete capsulectomy is warranted. The reality is that removal of the capsule may be quite difficult in the confined space of the calf and may require larger, unsightly incisions in more severe cases.

Major motor or sensory nerve injury in calf augmentation procedures is rare as the majority of dissection is performed in areas devoid of major neurovascular structures. It is quite common for patients to complain of some numbness over the area of the popliteal fossa postoperatively; however, this returns within 1 to 3 months postoperatively. Major motor and sensory deficits,

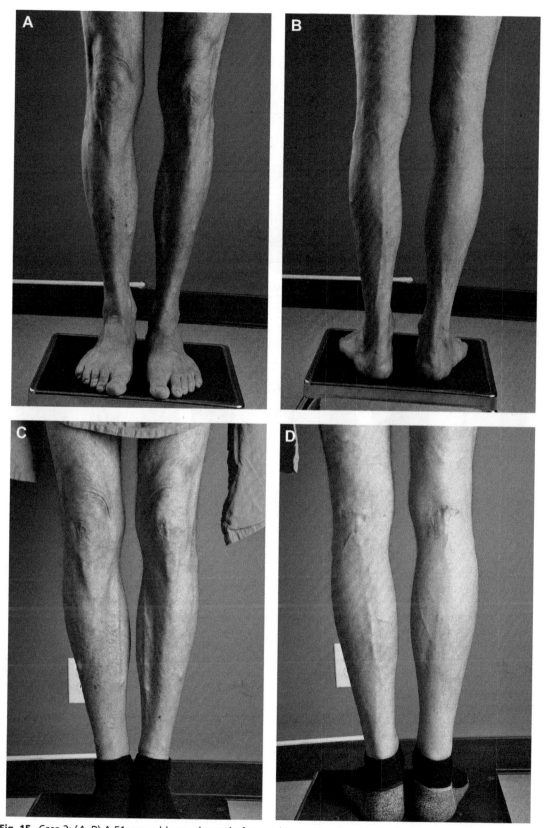

Fig. 15. Case 2: (*A–D*) A 51-year-old man shown before and 9 months after bilateral calf augmentation with style 2, size 2 implants.

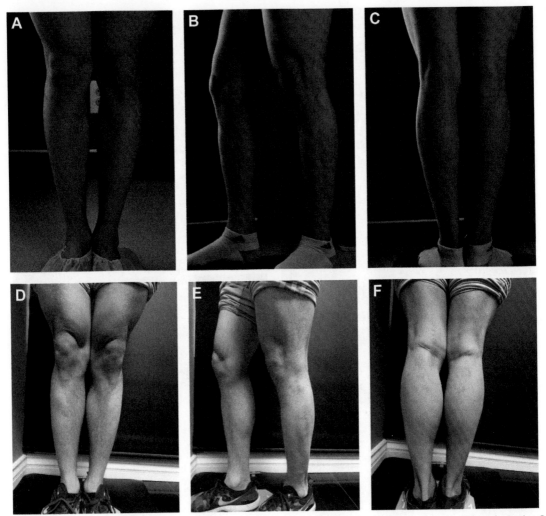

Fig. 16. Case 3: (A–F) A 29-year-old man before and 1 year after bilateral calf augmentation with style 2, size 2 implants.

particularly in the first 24 to 72 hours after surgery, can accompany compartment syndrome and this must be ruled out immediately if any significant deficits are appreciated. Compartment syndromes, typically seen in trauma, involve an acute increase in pressure inside a closed space, thereby impairing blood flow to the affected space and potentially putting the limb at risk for loss. Clinical signs of compartment syndrome include the 6 P's: pain, poikilothermia, pallor, paresthesias, paralysis, and pulselessness. In conscious patients, pain out of proportion to examination is the prominent symptom. Pain with passive range of motion is particularly troubling. In the lower extremity, numbness between the first and second toes due to compression of the deep peroneal nerve in the anterior compartment is the hallmark of early compartment syndrome. Progression to paralysis can occur, and loss of pulses is a late

sign. By the time pulselessness has occurred, it may be too late for limb salvage. In patients with a compatible history and a tense extremity, a clinical diagnosis may be sufficient. If the diagnosis is in doubt, compartment pressures may be measured with a hand-held Stryker device. An absolute pressure greater than 30 mm Hg in any compartment, or a pressure within 30 mm Hg of the diastolic blood pressure in hypotensive patients, or a patient with a concerning history who demonstrates the constellation of signs and symptoms of compartment syndrome are all possible indications for surgical compartment release via fasciotomy[17]; or, in the case of calf augmentation, simply opening the wound and removing the offending agent. In the case of calf augmentation, the cause of compartment syndrome is typically due to placing too large an implant in too small a space, thereby increasing the compartment

Box 1

Potential complications of calf augmentation surgery

- Infection
- Seroma
- Hematoma
- Asymmetry
- Implant visibility
- Hypertrophic scarring
- Hyperpigmentation of the scar
- Wound dehiscence
- Capsular contracture
- Nerve injury (permanent or temporary; motor or sensory)
- Compartment syndrome

Data from Chugay PN. Chapter 35: Calf Augmentation. In: Steinbrech, DS, ed. Male Aesthetic Plastic Surgery. 1st ed. Thieme; 2020. p. 419-434

pressure and causing arterial insufficiency or venous outflow compromise. This has been seen in the author's experience particularly in treating hypoplastic extremities, as seen in club foot deformity. Because the patient is postoperative, there is an implant in place and postoperative edema is present. Therefore, diagnosis may be problematic. In an affected compartment, accurate pressure readings may be difficult to obtain and may be inaccurate because of the patient's postoperative state. Clinical assessment and clinical diagnosis is the mainstay in compartment syndrome in the postoperative calf patient. Patients who are suspected of having compartment syndrome should have serial neurovascular checks and any worsening of the patient's examination warrants surgical intervention. A patient who is clinically stable has evidence of decreased pain or clinical improvement, and is cooperative may be a candidate for further close observation and neurovascular monitoring rather than immediate surgical intervention.[18]

Although the vast majority of patients presenting for calf augmentation are seeking increased

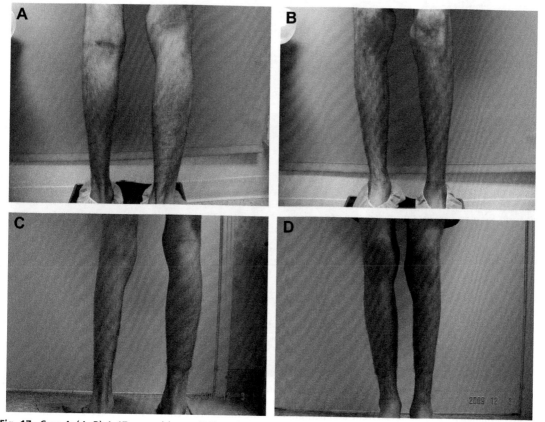

Fig. 17. Case 4: (*A–D*) A 17-year-old man (BC) underwent unilateral calf augmentation for a hypoplastic left calf (style 2, size 1).

muscularity, treatment of the hypoplastic leg is something that bears discussion. In patients that have been afflicted with club foot, polio, or trauma, there is at times a noticeable discrepancy in the size of the lower extremities. For those patients wishing to achieve symmetry, a calf implant may be an ideal way to do so (**Fig. 17**). However, that being said, a single augmentation may be insufficient to achieve symmetry. Lloyd Carlsen, knowing this full well, designed a custom expander to slowly expand the calf region without having to subject the patient to multiple operations and risk possible issues of skin slough and excessively elevated compartment pressures.[15,16] Although the idea of an expander makes sense, many patients are unwilling to go through a prolonged expansion period, as is commonly seen in breast patients postmastectomy reconstruction. It has been my standard practice to place a moderate-sized silicone prosthesis into position

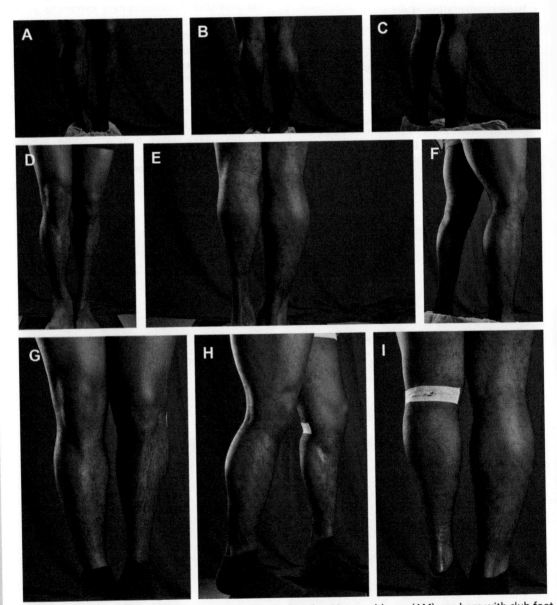

Fig. 18. Case 5: Staged procedures for calf augmentation. (*A–I*) A 30-year-old man (AM) was born with club foot deformity of the left leg. He presented for improved symmetry. He agreed to a staged procedure to bring about greater symmetry. First, he underwent augmentation of the medial calf with a style 2, size 2 implant. Subsequently, 8 months later, he underwent lateral calf augmentation with a style 3, size 1 implant. The next step will be either increasing the size of one of the implants or fat grafting to the lower leg, above the ankle.

as per the technique described previously. Then 6 months later, after having stretched out the proposed implant pocket, a second procedure can be performed with either a larger standard implant or a custom-made implant. Regardless of the second operation performed, the patient is able to enjoy a fairly normal lifestyle free of return doctor visits for expansion and the possible discomfort associated with uncomfortable ports. Although this method does require close attention in the postoperative period on the part of the patient and physician, it has been the author's experience that patients are much more content with the idea of this approach than the concept of slow expansion over time (**Fig. 18**).

CALF AUGMENTATION UTILIZING FAT INSTEAD OF IMPLANTS

One cannot have a thorough discussion of calf augmentation without mentioning the concept of fat grafting to the calf. Over the course of the development of the calf augmentation procedure, some physicians have begun to explore the use of fat grafting to correct hypoplastic calves.[19–21] The use of fat injection for augmentation was explored to eliminate some of the common complications associated with implants: implant palpability, lack of correction of the ankle region, implant displacement, and the possibility of capsular contracture. Erol's study of 2007 looked at 77 patients treated over a 10-year period with autologous fat and tissue cocktail injections, consisting of mini-micro grafts of dermis, fascia, and fat. They noted a moderate improvement in 13% of patients and a good improvement in 87% of patients. 75 to 200 cc of fat or tissue cocktail was injected into each leg to achieve the results noted in their study. These injections were repeated 2 to 4 times at 3-month intervals as was deemed necessary by the investigating physician. Although some surgeons swear by fat grafting and the use of a "natural" means of augmentation, I have found that fat grafting, specifically to the calf, does not always produce reliably pleasing results. The largest complaint typically noted in the author's fat grafting population is that the overall augmentation is not to their satisfaction or that the augmentation is asymmetric. These complaints are largely due to the variability in fat take and the potential for fat cell death. In the hands of many cosmetic surgeons, the average patient can expect a fat take of 50% to 70% without the use of stem cells.[22–26] However, this is largely dependent on placement of the fat in a place that has a rich blood supply that can foster the growth of the fat cells. When grafting to the calf,

the calf muscles are already largely hypoplastic and so there is a lack of a robust blood supply to support fat cell take, in our opinion. This being said, fat is a natural option for those seeking augmentation without implants. The surgeon must be careful to explain variable fat take and the possible need for further fat transfers to achieve symmetry or achieve more prominent augmentation.

SUMMARY

Calf augmentation with silicone implants is a procedure that can nicely enhance the physique of the male cosmetic patient in a reliable fashion and has a short learning curve. Overall patient satisfaction is quite high and can provide added volume medially, laterally, or to the overall calf region depending on the needs/desires of the patient.

CLINICS CARE POINTS

- Ensuring realistic expectations for calf augmentation patients is paramount to having good results and having happy patients.
- Choose the right implant for every patient based on patient desires and established esthetic norms
- Careful and judicious dissection is the key to avoiding complications intraoperatively and postoperatively.
- Layered closure with absorbable sutures ensures a more esthetically pleasing scar postoperatively.
- Compression, compression, compression .... Wrap for compression in the first 24 hours to minimize implant mobility and keep swelling compartmentalized is an early intervention that is key to success. Postoperative use of compression stockings with a grading of 20 to 30 mm Hg helps to minimize the dead space and the risk of implant movement until scar tissue has developed.

DISCLOSURE

The author has nothing to disclose.

REFERENCES

1. Aiache AE. Calf implantation. Plast Reconstr Surg 1989;83:488.
2. Dini M, Innocenti A, Lorenzetti P. Aesthetic calf augmentation with silicone implants. Aesthetic Plast Surg 2002;26:490.

3. Howard PS. Calf augmentation and correction of contour deformities. Clin Plast Surg 1991;18: 601.

4. Szalay LV. Twelve years' experience of calf augmentation. Aesthetic Plast Surg 1995;19:473.

5. Niechajev I. Calf augmentation and restoration. Plast Reconstr Surg 2005;116:295.

6. Kalixto MA, Vergara R. Submuscular calf implants. Aesthet Plast. Surg. 2003;27:135.

7. Gutstein RA. Augmentation of the lower leg: a new combined calf-tibial implant. Plast Reconstr Surg 2006;117:817–26.

8. Nunes GO, Garcia DP. Calf Augmentation with supraperiostic solid prosthesis associated with fasciotomies. Aesthetic Plast Surg 2004;28:17.

9. Gray H. Anatomy of the human body. Philadelphia (PA): Lea & Febiger; 1918.

10.. Chugay P, Chugay N. Calf augmentation: a single institution review of over 200 cases. Am J Cosmet Surg 2013;30(2):64–71.

11. De la Pena-Salcedo JA, Soto-Miranda MA, Lopez-Salguero JF. Calf Implants: a 25 year experience and an anatomical review. Aesthetic Plast Surg 2012;36:261–70.

12. Aiache AE. Calf contour correction with implants. Clin Plast Surg 1991;18:857–62.

13. Carlsen LN. Calf augmentation: a preliminary report. Ann Plast Surg 1979;2:508.

14. Glitzenstein J. Correction of the amyotrophies of the limbs with silicone prosthesis inclusions. Rev Bras Cir 1979;69:117.

15. Carlsen LN, Voice SD. Calf augmentation. In: Vistnes LM, editor. Boston: Little Brown: Procedures in plastic surgery: how they do it, chapter 15; 1991. p. 281–94.

16. Carlsen LN. Calf augmentation. Operative Techniques in Plastic and Reconstructive Surgery 1996; 3(2):145–53.

17. Cothren CC, Biffl WL, Moore EE. Chapter 7. Trauma. In: Brunicardi FC, Andersen DK, Billiar TR, et al, editors. Schwartz's Principles of Surgery, 9e. McGraw Hill; 2010.

18. Walsh J, Page S. Chapter 10. Rhabdomyolysis and Compartment Syndrome in Military Trainees. In Recruit Medicine.

19. Erol OO, Gürlek A, Agaoglu G, et al. Calf augmentation with autologous tissue injection. Plast Reconstr Surg 2008;6:121.

20. Veber M Jr, Mojallal A. Calf augmentation with autologous tissue injection. Plast Reconst Surg 2010;125: 423–4.

21. Hendy A. Calf and leg augmentation: autologous fat or silicone implant? J Plast Reconst Surg 2010; 34(2):123–6.

22. Coleman SR. Long-term survival of fat transplants: controlled demonstrations. Aesthetic Plast Surg 1995;19:421.

23. Coleman SR. Structureal fat grafts: the ideal filler? Clin Plast Surg 2001;28:111.

24. Pereira LH, Nicaretta B, Sterodimas A. Bilateral calf augmentation for aesthetic purposes. Aesthetic Plast Surg 2012;36:295–302.

25. Sterodimas A, de Faria J, Correa WE, et al. Tissue engineering in plastic surgery: an up to date review of the current literature. Ann Plast Surg 2009;62: 97–103.

26. Sterodimas A, de Faria J, Nicaretta B, et al. Tissue engineering with adipose-derive stem cells: current and future applications. J Plast Reconstr Aesthet Surg 2010;63(11):1886–92.

The Role of Energy-Based Devices in Male Body Contouring

Darren M. Smith, MD

KEYWORDS

- Male body contouring • Minimally invasive body contouring • BodyTite • Emsculpt Neo
- Radiofrequency energy • HIFEM

KEY POINTS

- Energy-based devices can extend the indications of minimally invasive body contouring procedures in men.
- Patient selection and education are key in realizing success with these modalities.
- Energy-based devices cannot be expected to replicate the results of more invasive procedures.
- Combining energy-based devices can often yield the best results.

BACKGROUND

Body contouring procedures can be conceptualized as having 2 components: adjustment of tissue volume and the fitting of overlying skin to that adjusted volume. Liposuction allows us to control tissue volume and thus anatomic shape quite effectively with minimal scar burden. In young, healthy patients with excellent skin elasticity, the skin will generally contract to fit the newly sculpted form. In older patients or those with less elastic skin for other reasons, skin contraction is less reliable. In these patients, the most stunning volumetric contouring might be completely obscured by a loose skin envelope. It is in these cases that skin excision becomes necessary to achieve desirable results. The great trade-off in skin excision procedures, however, has always been the removal of skin excess in exchange for scars. The greater the magnitude of skin excision, the longer the necessary scar. The introduction of energy-based devices has allowed us to shift this calculus. By inducing skin and soft tissue contraction with energy in the form of heat, we can see better-defined results by augmenting skin elasticity in those with varying degrees of skin laxity. Energy-based devices have further extended our body contouring capabilities by allowing for the noninvasive destruction of fat as well as the induction of muscle growth. The advent of energy-based devices is particularly relevant to male body contouring, as plastic surgery and aesthetic medicine for men are subject to a relatively greater taboo. While this taboo is fading, the prospect of attaining significant results with minimal or no scars and downtime is making these procedures more approachable for men. Here, we will begin by reviewing the state of the art in energy-based devices frequently in use for male body contouring and proceed into a practical discussion of methods for success with these devices by anatomic area.

DISCUSSION

There is a wide array of energy-based devices presently available, and this selection seems to increase by the month. This ever-growing assortment implies that first, these devices show great promise, and second, that no one device has yet emerged as a clearly dominant solution. For the purposes of our discussion, we can separate these devices into minimally invasive modalities (which tend to have more significant effects) and noninvasive modalities (whose results tend to be less profound). We will then focus on devices in

111 East 57th, Street, Suite 1.1, New York, NY 10022, USA
E-mail address: dmsmith@darrensmithmd.com

Clin Plastic Surg 49 (2022) 329–337
https://doi.org/10.1016/j.cps.2022.01.001
0094-1298/22/© 2022 Elsevier Inc. All rights reserved.

each category that the author finds to be instructive examples. It is intended that this discussion will serve as a framework that can be generalized to a broader exploration of present devices and future modalities as they become available.

We will begin with minimally invasive devices, as they comprise the cornerstone of energy-based surgery. Minimally invasive energy-based body contouring devices are passed through the same ports used for liposuction, so no additional scarring is necessary. We regularly use 2 forms of a minimally invasive energy-based device in our practice. The first is a bipolar radiofrequency energy device, BodyTite, which targets superficial connective tissues and dermis. This treatment is designed to "shrink wrap" the skin envelope to contour achieved with liposuction. The second device, VASER, uses ultrasound energy to tighten deeper tissues, potentiating the volumetric changes achieved with liposuction. VASER offers some skin tightening benefits as well. We will then discuss a representative noninvasive device, Emsculpt Neo. Emsculpt Neo combines electromagnetic energy for muscle building with radiofrequency energy for fat destruction. Emsculpt Neo can be combined with minimally invasive body contouring procedures or performed independently.

BodyTite

Radiofrequency energy saw its first clinical use in the form of electrocautery in the 1920s, has been used extensively for collagen contraction (eg, tightening loose ligaments) in orthopedics, and is now increasing in popularity in plastic surgery since its introduction into aesthetics by Thermage in 2002.[1–4] Minimally invasive energy-based devices like BodyTite offer a solution to those patients that will not see sufficient soft tissue contraction with liposuction alone but who may not require (or are averse to undergoing) classic excisional skin procedures.[5] Dayan clearly reviewed the mechanism for tissue contraction in response to radiofrequency energy as follows.[3] Radiofrequency energy generates heat in tissue due to the target tissue's resistance to the passage of electromagnetic current. The heat generated by radiofrequency energy causes soft tissue contraction by 2 mechanisms. First, in an immediate effect, the hydrogen bonds in collagen's triple helix are cleaved, yielding shorter, thicker collagen fibrils. Second, a wound healing cascade is triggered that, over the ensuing 3 to 4 months yields neocollagenesis, elastin reorganization, and neoangiogenesis. From a practical standpoint, optimal tissue contraction is obtained at skin

surface temperatures from 38°C to 42°C and subdermal temperatures from 65°C to 68°C.

Radiofrequency energy can be delivered for the purpose of soft tissue tightening in several forms (monopolar, bipolar, and multipolar), and several devices have evolved to capitalize on each of these modalities. We have seen the best balance of high-quality results and an excellent safety profile with bipolar radiofrequency energy (BodyTite), so this device will be our focus here. The BodyTite device has one pole that is inserted into the subdermal tissue and another pole that follows along extracorporeally, effectively "sandwiching" the target tissue between the 2 poles [**Fig. 1**]. Each of the poles contains a thermistor (a resistor whose level of resistance is determined by temperature) allowing for very precise control of the temperature in the intervening tissue between the 2 poles. The internal pole is bullet-shaped to facilitate its movement through tissue while minimizing the risk of end-hits (delivery of dangerous levels of thermal energy to superficial tissues).[6] This pole is positively charged and emits ablative, coagulative energy that liquefies fat and causes contraction of horizontal, vertical and oblique fibers of the fibroseptal network. This energy travels to the external negatively charged electrode which tightens the papillary and reticular dermis in a nonablative manner.[7–9] Greater than 25% soft tissue area reduction has been shown at 6 months after BodyTite with an increase to 34% after 12 months.[10]

We nearly always perform BodyTite in conjunction with liposuction [**Fig. 2**]. Even in cases whereby we are not aiming to reduce adipose volume, a small amount of fat is liquefied and rendered unviable by the BodyTite device. In these cases, a minimal amount of suction is performed to extract this liquefied adipose tissue and as little unaffected fat as possible. In most cases, however, some degree of fat removal is indicated. Therefore, these cases should be set up in the same manner as one is accustomed to preparing for liposuction cases. Following this theme, limited BodyTite procedures encompassing only a small surface area can reasonably be performed with local anesthesia and varying degrees of oral anxiolysis.[11] Larger cases should be performed with IV sedation or general anesthesia.

The first step of the BodyTite procedure is the instillation of tumescent solution into the treatment area, just as one would do for liposuction. Whether most of the liposuction is performed before or after BodyTite is a matter of personal preference. While performing liposuction first is theoretically time-saving (less tissue is present in the treatment area so goal temperature can be reached more

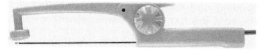

Fig. 1. The BodyTite handpiece is shown, illustrating the smaller internal pole and larger external probe. (*Courtesy of* InMode, Irvine, CA.)

rapidly), the decreased volume of fat may render the treatment area more vulnerable to thermal injury. If one does decide to perform liposuction before BodyTite, it is advisable to perform a pass of low volume suction after BodyTite to remove any fat liquefied by the radiofrequency energy. It is our preference to perform BodyTite first and follow this with suction-assisted lipectomy.

Results with BodyTite are fairly operator dependent. Here we outline the points we feel are key for success with this device. When performing BodyTite, we recommend separating the treatment area into smaller subsections and sequentially treating each section to completion before moving on. In this manner, goal temperature can be reached most efficiently. "Completion" is achieved when the goal temperature is met and sustained for several minutes. There are 3 popular methods of delivering energy with the BodyTite device: retrograde, bidirectional, and stamping. In retrograde energy delivery, the device is inserted to the maximum planned length and energy is delivered as the device is withdrawn. In bidirectional energy delivery, the device is activated on both insertion and removal. In stamping, the device is inserted to target a specific point and energy is delivered. It is then moved to the next point and more energy is delivered as a discrete action. This process is repeated until the entire treatment area is treated to completion. The

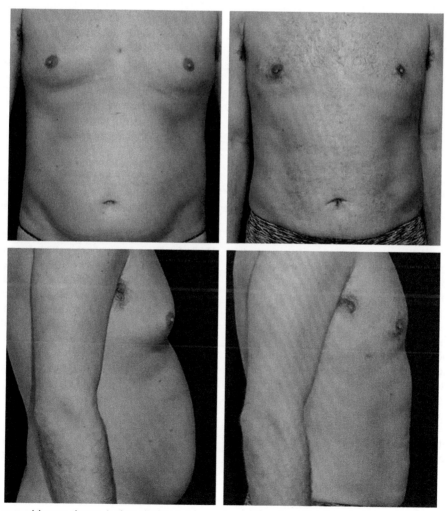

Fig. 2. 35-year-old man shown before (*left*) and several months after (*right*) BodyTite and liposuction of the chest, abdomen, and waist, as well as direct excision of breast tissue.

bidirectional method is the most efficient and our method of choice due to its efficiency. There is, however, a higher risk of end hits with resulting thermal injury on anterograde strokes, so in more topographically challenging regions we may revert to the more conservative, though slower, retrograde approach. In our practice, stamping is reserved for hard-to-reach points that cannot be easily incorporated into a bidirectional or retrograde stroke. It is worth noting that more rapid strokes tend to favor superficial heating and slower strokes tend to favor deeper heating. Speed is modulated to differentially heat superficial or deep tissue as needed to reach the goal temperature of each.

VASER

Zocchi introduced ultrasound-assisted liposuction as a method to selectively target adipose tissue for less traumatic, more efficient removal while sparing neurovascular structures.[12] This has evolved into the VASER (vibration amplification of sound energy at resonance) in use today, which uses titanium rods of varying lengths and diameters to transmit ultrasound energy to the treatment area. The distal tip of the VASER probe is encircled by a varying number of grooves designed to transmit the ultrasound energy into the target tissue. A larger number of grooves yields more robust tissue fragmentation while a smaller number of grooves favors improved tissue penetration.[13]

The ultrasound energy emitted from the VASER probe is clinically useful due to cavitation. Schafer offers an excellent description of the basics of cavitation.[14] We can summarize here as follows. Microbubbles of air unavoidably diffuse into tumescent solution at room temperature and atmospheric pressure. As fat cells are only loosely packed together (to allow for significant volume fluctuation with lipid storage requirements), these microbubbles can wedge themselves between fat cells as tumescent solution is infiltrated into the treatment area. Conversely, the cells of other tissue types in the treatment area (eg, vascular, muscle, connective tissue) are much more firmly adherent to one another and do not allow for the interposition of microbubbles. When subjected to the ultrasound field emitted by the VASER probe, the air bubbles sequentially grow and collapse. This agitation frees the adipocytes from the surrounding connective tissue matrix, facilitating their extraction in the subsequent suction step. VASER technology facilitates fat removal, protects vascular structures, and enhances aesthetic outcomes.[15,16] It also yields significantly less blood loss than traditional liposuction, with Garcia reporting 7.5 times lower hemoglobin of the aspirate from the former as compared with aspirate from the latter.[17]

It is advisable to perform all but small volume VASER liposuction procedures under IV sedation or general anesthesia. This guidance maximizes patient safety, enhances the quality of the results that can be achieved, and optimizes patient comfort. These cases should be set up essentially following existing practices for tumescent liposuction cases. The general order of events is the infiltration of tumescent solution into the treatment area, allowing sufficient time for the tumescent to act, treatment of the tissue with the VASER device, and finally, suction-assisted lipectomy.

Specific considerations regarding the VASER device are as follows. Access incisions may need to be slightly larger than typically made for liposuction to accommodate skin protectors. These are affixed to the access incisions with either staples or sutures to shield the skin edges from the heat generated by the device. We also like to protect the access points with a saline-soaked lap sponge during VASER treatment. VASER probes are available in a range of dimensions and tip ring configurations. We find that the 3.7 mm three-ring tip is our workhorse probe with broad applications throughout the body. The intensity of the treatment can be set in 10% increments from 0 to 100. We generally find 70% to achieve excellent results without exposing the tissue to undue levels of thermal energy. The device may be operated in either a continuous energy delivery mode or a pulsed energy delivery mode. We use the pulsed mode almost exclusively as we are able to achieve excellent results in this manner while substantially reducing energy exposure and associated risk. While traditional guidelines calling for 1 minute of VASER treatment time per 100 cc of tumescent fluid have been called outdated[18] as this degree of VASER is often not necessary to achieve the desired result, we find this maxim to offer a useful safety limit. In practice, we treat the target area until minimal tissue resistance remains, and this endpoint is generally reached in significantly less time than 1 minute per 100 cc of tumescent fluid used.

EMSCULPT NEO

Noninvasive body contouring has been wildly popular since its introduction. The promise of improved body shape and muscle definition without surgery or downtime is understandably alluring. These technologies first focused on fat reduction with either heat or cold-induced adipocyte destruction. In 2018, the first device targeted at muscle development (Emsculpt) came to market. Emsculpt used HIFEM (high intensity focused electromagnetic energy) to force involuntary muscle contractions, yielding myocyte hypertrophy and hyperplasia. In addition to yielding muscle growth, HIFEM was found to trigger some degree of fat reduction. Most interestingly, HIFEM was shown to decrease visceral fat by 14.3%.[19] For some time, noninvasive fat destruction devices were used in series with muscle-building devices to achieve fat reduction and improved muscle definition in the treatment area. In an effort to increase efficiency for patients and providers, attention was focused on developing devices that could simultaneously destroy fat and build muscle. The first such device, Emsculpt Neo, came to market in 2020. Emsculpt Neo combines alternating pulses of HIFEM and radiofrequency energy to simultaneously build muscle with the former and destroy fat with the latter. The combination of HIFEM and radiofrequency energy proved quite effective, yielding an average 30.8% fat reduction and 26.1% muscle thickening by MRI.[20] Corroborating histology demonstrated a 30.2% increase in skeletal muscle satellite cells as well as adipocyte shrinkage (31.7%) and apoptosis.[21,22]

Emsculpt Neo is FDA cleared for use on multiple body areas. The abdomen [**Fig. 3**] and buttocks are the most common treatment sites. Of note, the treatment program for the buttocks is designed for muscle growth with minimized fat loss, as the intention in this area is to achieve a lift and volume increase. Other FDA-cleared areas include the biceps, triceps, circumferential thigh, and calf. The recommended treatment regimen includes 4 sessions that are 30 minutes each, separated by 1 week. While skin tightening is not an FDA-cleared indication, we have seen evidence of skin tightening in our practice. This is consistent with the expected tissue effects associated with the temperatures reached with the radiofrequency energy.

We use Emsculpt Neo both as a standalone treatment and in combination with minimally invasive body contouring procedures. When used alone, we find the device will offer pleasing results to properly selected patients that are educated to have reasonable expectations. It must be made very clear to patients that this treatment is not a substitute for liposuction or other surgery, but real improvements can be expected. There is a risk, as with any noninvasive treatment, of under-response. This however is the exception, and most patients are quite satisfied. We describe predicted results as getting patients "to the next level" of body contour. For example, someone with significant abdominal adiposity can expect to see a reduction, but they certainly will not have a flat abdomen with muscle definition. Alternatively, someone with minimal abdominal adiposity but without muscle definition can expect to have some definition after treatment. Finally, someone with early muscle definition will likely see that definition significantly increased after treatment [**Fig. 4**].

Emsculpt Neo can also be used to enhance the results of minimally invasive body contouring procedures. In these instances, we like to wait at least 2 weeks after the initial procedure to begin treatment with Emsculpt Neo to allow for initial healing and to permit the return of some protective sensation to the region. One rare risk of Emsculpt Neo is thermal injury, and reduced sensation can increase this risk.

REGIONAL STRATEGIES
Abdomen and waist

The abdomen and waist are the 2 areas men are most interested in contouring in our practice. While some may be interested in contouring one of these areas and not the other, it is almost always beneficial to treat both areas together to achieve ideal proportions. In contouring the male torso, we are aiming to highlight naturally existing landmarks from the front (eg, semilunar lines) and a V-shape is achieved from the posterior perspective. We find that VASER is very useful in achieving deep tissue contraction in men with significant superficial abdominal adiposity. It also facilitates suction-assisted lipectomy in the fibrous tissue of the back and posterior waist. VASER can be used more superficially in the context of high definition liposuction (see Mentz's early descriptions of abdominal etching[23,24] that have been amended to include VASER as techniques popularized by Hoyos).[16,25]

Ultrasound energy has also been combined with abdominoplasty to enhance this procedure. Davidson described using the Mentor Contour Genesis ultrasound machine to treat the abdominoplasty flap overlying but not lateral to the rectus sheath, citing decreased local tissue trauma as compared with standard liposuction, which is of course of paramount concern when suctioning this potentially sensitive region.[26] Hoyos described more extensive suction of the flap as well as the incorporation of circumferential liposuction with third-generation ultrasound assistance (VASER). This approach allowed him to achieve improved waistline definition and enhanced flap aesthetics.[15]

BodyTite is useful for superficial soft tissue tightening in the abdomen of men who may be on the

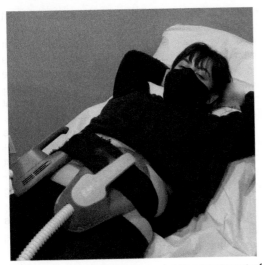

Fig. 3. Patient undergoing Emsculpt Neo treatment of the abdomen.

We strongly encourage all abdomen and flank liposuction patients to undergo a series of Emsculpt Neo treatments after their surgery. We find that in addition to the benefits described earlier, the process accelerates the resolution of edema and the manifestation of contour improvement.

Chest

In considering an appropriate treatment plan for gynecomastia, the first practical concern is whether enough glandular tissue is present in addition to excess adiposity to warrant direct excision along with a suction-based strategy. We will almost never perform skin excision as part of the primary operation as all but the most severe cases will, after several months, demonstrate sufficient skin contraction to avoid the stigmata of skin excision. In cases for which we are particularly concerned about skin excess, we will incorporate BodyTite into our primary procedure. It is our preference to use VASER in all gynecomastia cases, for 3 reasons. First, the adipose tissue of the male breast is quite fibrous, and the incorporation of VASER can consistently enhance the efficacy and decrease the trauma of suction-assisted lipectomy in this context. Second, the ultrasound energy contributes to enhanced contraction of the soft tissue envelope and therefore overall cosmetic result. Third, while we do not find that VASER can be relied on to sufficiently fragment glandular tissue to a degree that precludes the need for resection, it is possible that in cases on the border of requiring glandular excision, VASER disrupts the stromal tissue sufficiently to obviate this step. In cases with significant glandular tissue, this can be excised per the surgeon's preferred protocol after adipose reduction with VASER-

verge of requiring an abdominoplasty to achieve an aesthetically pleasing result. Especially when combined with VASER, sufficient soft tissue and skin tightening can often, in our experience, be achieved in these borderline cases to achieve satisfactory cosmesis without the scars of formal abdominoplasty. It is critical in these cases to discuss expectations with the patient and educate him that he will not achieve abdominoplasty-like results with this procedure, but dramatic improvement may be possible, nonetheless. It is advisable to also walk these patients through the abdominoplasty process and assess their willingness to consider it as a lifeboat option should a disagreeable amount of skin excess remain after their procedure.

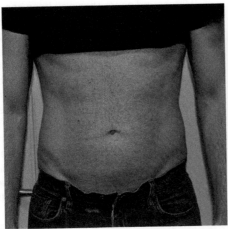
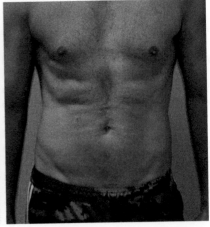

Fig. 4. 52-year-old man shown before (*left*) and several months after (*right*) Emsculpt Neo of the abdomen.

assisted liposuction.[27] See also Hoyos's expansion of the concept of using VASER to debulk the male chest into a framework for achieving enhanced definition of this region.[28]

Arms

We consider the arms as having 2 compartments that are primarily amenable to minimally invasive contouring after Theodorou and Chia: the deltoid fat pad and the triceps fat pad.[29] VASER and BodyTite have both proved to be useful adjuncts to suction-assisted lipectomy of the triceps fat pad, as there is significant potential for skin and deeper soft tissue laxity in this region. We rarely use VASER, and almost never BodyTite, when treating the deltoid fat pad as soft tissue laxity is seldom a concern in this area. Hunstad group reports that of the various energy-based devices they have used, VASER has been the most efficacious in their experience for achieving soft tissue tightening of the arms.[30] We have also found BodyTite to be a very effective modality in patients with significant skin laxity in the triceps region, allowing for substantial skin tightening without the stigmata of formal brachioplasty. Indeed, Duncan reported a mean surface area reduction of 33.5% and a shortening of vertical hang of 50% in her series for this region.[31]

More severe cases, particularly those presenting with skin laxity after massive weight loss, may only find successful resolution of their concerns with brachioplasty. Liposuction has been combined with brachioplasty for some time[32,33] in an effort to improve aesthetic outcomes, reduce or eliminate the need for undermining, reduce or eliminate the creation of dead space, and subsequently reduce the rate of seroma formation and wound healing problems. The addition of VASER to the liposuction portion of these procedures[34] can potentiate all these effects by tightening skin and soft tissue and reducing the trauma with which the suction-assisted lipectomy is performed.

Thighs

Lockwood popularized the medial thigh lift incorporating liposuction, undermining, and soft tissue excision and highlighted the importance of deep fascial anchoring to offload tension from the incision line and preserve the aesthetic result.[34–36] As with the VASER-assisted brachioplasty, the addition of VASER to the liposuction portion of a medial thigh lift can both enhance the aesthetic outcome by improving tissue tone and decrease the risk of complications by decreasing trauma to the tissues involved.[34] Additionally, in borderline cases, the combined use of VASER for deep tissue

laxity and BodyTite for sagging skin may obviate the need for thigh lift altogether.

SUMMARY

Male body contouring procedures are rapidly growing in popularity. Noninvasive modalities offer the possibility of improved contour to those who may never have considered even a minimally invasive operation. Moreover, the thoughtful application of energy-based devices can not only enhance the results possible with classic minimally invasive procedures but also extend the indications of these procedures. In properly selected patients, these devices may obviate the need for more invasive approaches by contracting skin and deeper soft tissues to avoid tissue excision and its resultant tell-tale scarring. We have reviewed the landscape of energy-based devices that are useful in male body contouring procedures as it exists today and discussed our framework for considering the use of these devices. We have advanced the hypothesis that the best approach is often a combined approach.[37] With careful attention to patient selection and patient education, the results that are possible with energy-based modalities offer an exciting new dimension to male body contouring.

CLINICS CARE POINTS

- Energy-based devices can extend the indications of minimally invasive procedures in male body contouring by tightening skin and soft tissues.

- VASER uses ultrasound energy mediated by cavitation to selectively fragment adipose tissue and tighten deep connective tissue and skin.

- BodyTite uses bipolar radiofrequency energy to tighten the fibroseptal network and dermis.

- Emsculpt Neo combines HIFEM and radiofrequency energy to simultaneously build muscle and destroy fat.

- Patient selection and expectation management is essential to success with energy-based devices in male body contouring.

- Often a combination of minimally invasive and noninvasive procedures will yield the best results.

DISCLOSURE

The authors have nothing to disclose.

REFERENCES

1. Alexiades-Armenakas M, Dover JS. Unipolar versus bipolar radiofrequency treatment of rhytides and laxity using a mobile painless delivery method. Lasers Surg Med 2008;446–53.
2. Miniaci A, Codsi MJ. Thermal capsulorrhaphy for the treatment of shoulder instability. Am J Sports Med 2006;34:1356–63.
3. Dayan E, Burns AJ, Rohrich RJ. The use of radiofrequency in aesthetic surgery. Plast Surg Glob Open 2020;1–6.
4. Fisher GH, Jacobson LG, Bernstein LJ, et al. Nonablative radiofrequency treatment of facial laxity. Dermatol Surg 2005;31:1237–41.
5. Theodorou SJ, Vecchio DD. Soft tissue contraction in body contouring with radiofrequency-assisted liposuction: a treatment gap solution. Aesthet Surg J 2018;S75–83.
6. Mulholland RS. BodyTite®: the Science and art of radiofrequency assisted Lipocoagulation (RFAL) in body contouring surgery. The art of body contouring. IntechOpen 2019. Available at: https://www.intechopen.com/chapters/65219.
7. Mulholland RS. Internal and External Radiofrequency Assisted Lipo-Coagulation (RFAL) in the control of soft tissue contraction during liposuction: Part 1 "inside Out" thermal tissue tightening. Enhanced Liposuction - New Perspect Tech 2021. IntechOpen Available at: https://www.intechopen.com/online-first/76342.
8. Paul M, Blugerman G, Kreindel M, et al. Three-dimensional radiofrequency tissue tightening: a proposed mechanism and applications for body contouring. Aesthetic Plast Surg 2011;35:87–95.
9. Kreindel M, Mulholland S. The basic Science of radiofrequency-based devices. Enhanced Liposuction-New Perspect Tech 2021. IntechOpen Available at: https://www.intechopen.com/online-first/76342https://www.intechopen.com/online-first/75578.
10. Duncan DI. Nonexcisional tissue tightening: creating skin surface area reduction during abdominal liposuction by adding radiofrequency heating. Aesthet Surg J 2013;33:1154–66.
11. Theodorou SJ, Paresi RJ, Chia CT. Radiofrequency-assisted liposuction device for body contouring: 97 patients under local anesthesia. Aesthetic Plast Surg 2012;767–79.
12. Zocchi M. Ultrasonic liposculpturing. Aesthetic Plast Surg 1992;16:287–98.
13. Beidas OE, Gusenoff JA. Update on liposuction: what all plastic surgeons should Know. Plast Reconstr Surg 2021;658e–68e.
14. Schafer ME. Basic Science of ultrasound in body contouring. Ultrasound-Assisted Liposuction 2020; 9–21.
15. Hoyos A, Perez ME, Guarin DE, et al. A report of 736 high-definition lipoabdominoplasties performed in conjunction with circumferential VASER liposuction. Plast Reconstr Surg 2018;142(3):662–75.
16. Hoyos AE, Millard JA. VASER-assisted high-definition liposculpture. Aesthet Surg J 2007; 594–604.
17. Garcia O Jr, Nathan N. Comparative analysis of blood loss in suction-assisted lipoplasty and third-generation internal ultrasound-assisted lipoplasty. Aesthet Surg J 2008;28:430–5.
18. Garcia O. Contouring of the Trunk. Ultrasound-assisted liposuction. Cham (Switzerland): Springer; 2020. p. 65–86.
19. Kent DE, Kinney BM. The effect of high-intensity focused electromagnetic procedure on visceral adipose tissue: Retrospective assessment of computed tomography scans. J Cosmet Dermatol 2021;20: 757–62.
20. Jacob C, Kent D, Ibrahim O. Efficacy and safety of simultaneous application of HIFEM and synchronized radiofrequency for abdominal fat reduction and muscle toning: a Multicenter Magnetic resonance Imaging Evaluation study. Dermatol Surg 2021;969–73.
21. Halaas Y, Duncan D, Bernardy J. Activation of skeletal muscle satellite cells by a device simultaneously applying high-intensity focused electromagnetic technology and novel RF technology: Fluorescent Microscopy Facilitated Detection of NCAM/CD56. Aesthet Surg J 2021;NP939–47.
22. Goldberg DJ. Deletion of adipocytes induced by a novel device simultaneously delivering synchronized radiofrequency and hifem: Human histological study. J Cosmet Dermatol 2021;1104–9.
23. Agochukwu-Nwubah N, Mentz HA. Abdominal etching: past and present. Aesthet Surg J 2019; 1368–77.
24. Mentz HA, Gilliland MD, Patronella CK. Abdominal etching: differential liposuction to detail abdominal musculature. Aesthetic Plast Surg 1993;17:287–90.
25. Hoyos AE, Guarin DE. High-definition body contouring using VASER-assisted liposuction. Ultrasound-Assisted Liposuction 2020;203–11.
26. Abramson DL. Ultrasound-assisted abdominoplasty: combining modalities in a safe and effective technique. Plast Reconstr Surg 2003;898–902.
27. Garcia O. VASER-assisted liposuction of gynecomastia. Ultrasound-assisted liposuction. Cham (Switzerland): Springer; 2020. p. 87–98.
28. Hoyos AE, Perez ME. Gynecomastia treatment through open resection and pectoral high-definition liposculpture. Plast Reconstr Surg 2021; 1072–83.

29. Theodorou S, Chia C. Radiofrequency-assisted lipo-suction for arm contouring: technique under local anesthesia. Plast Reconstr Surg Glob Open 2013; 1:1–13.

30. Vasilakis V, Isakson MH, Yamin F, et al. Four-position four-entry site circumferential arm liposuction: technique overview and experience. Aesthetic Plast Surg 2020;1596–603.

31. Duncan DI. Improving outcomes in upper arm lipo-suction: adding radiofrequency-assisted liposuction to induce skin contraction. Aesthet Surg J 2012;32: 84–95.

32. Hurwitz DJ, Holland SW. Brachioplasty with liposuc-tion resection. In: Rubin JP, Jewell ML, Richter DF, et al, editors. Body contouring and liposuction. Phil-adelphia: Saunders; 2013. p. 29–34.

33. Hurwitz DJ, Holland SW. The L brachioplasty: an innovative approach to correct excess tissue of the upper arm, axilla, and lateral chest. Plast Reconstr Surg 2006;117:403–11.

34. Garcia O. Contouring of the Extremities. Ultrasound-assisted liposuction. Cham (Switzerland): Springer; 2020. p. 99–132.

35. Lockwood T. Lower body lift with superficial fascial system suspension. Plast Reconstr Surg 1993;92: 1112–22.

36. Lockwood TE. Maximizing aesthetics in lateral-tension abdominoplasty and body lifts. Clin Plast Surg 2004;31:523–37.

37. Hurwitz DJ, Wright L. Noninvasive abdominoplasty. Clin Plast Surg 2020;379–88.

Moving?

Make sure your subscription moves with you!

To notify us of your new address, find your **Clinics Account Number** (located on your mailing label above your name), and contact customer service at:

Email: journalscustomerservice-usa@elsevier.com

800-654-2452 (subscribers in the U.S. & Canada)
314-447-8871 (subscribers outside of the U.S. & Canada)

Fax number: 314-447-8029

Elsevier Health Sciences Division
Subscription Customer Service
3251 Riverport Lane
Maryland Heights, MO 63043

*To ensure uninterrupted delivery of your subscription, please notify us at least 4 weeks in advance of move.

Printed and bound by CPI Group (UK) Ltd, Croydon, CR0 4YY

08/05/2025

01864713-0015